T0295107

Exotic Animal Practice Around the World

Editor

SHANGZHE XIE

VETERINARY CLINICS OF NORTH AMERICA: EXOTIC ANIMAL PRACTICE

www.vetexotic.theclinics.com

Consulting Editor
JÖRG MAYER

September 2024 • Volume 27 • Number 3

ELSEVIER

1600 John F. Kennedy Boulevard • Suite 1800 • Philadelphia, Pennsylvania, 19103-2899
http://www.vetexotic.theclinics.com

VETERINARY CLINICS OF NORTH AMERICA: EXOTIC ANIMAL PRACTICE Volume 27, Number 3
September 2024 ISSN 1094-9194, ISBN-13: 978-0-443-24662-3

Editor: Stacy Eastman
Developmental Editor: Varun Gopal

Veterinary Clinics of North America: Exotic Animal Practice (ISSN 1094-9194) is published in January, May, and September by Elsevier, Inc., 360 Park Avenue South, New York, NY 10010-1710. Subscription prices are $311.00 per year for US individuals, $100.00 per year for US students and residents, $362.00 per year for Canadian individuals, $377.00 per year for international individuals, $100.00 per year Canadian students/residents, and $165.00 per year for international students/residents. For institutional access pricing please contact Customer Service via the contact information below. To receive student/resident rate, orders must be accompanied by name of affiliated institution, date of term, and the *signature* of program/residency coordinator on institution letterhead. Orders will be billed at individual rate until proof of status is received. Foreign air speed delivery is included in all *Clinics* subscription prices. All prices are subject to change without notice. Orders, claims, and journal inquiries: Please visit our Support Hub page https://service.elsevier.com for assistance.

Reprints. For copies of 100 or more of articles in this publication, please contact the Commercial Reprints Department, Elsevier Inc., 360 Park Avenue South, New York, New York 10010-1710. Tel.: 212-633-3874; Fax: 212-633-3820; E-mail: reprints@elsevier.com.

Veterinary Clinics of North America: Exotic Animal Practice is covered in *MEDLINE/PubMed (Index Medicus)*.

Contributors

CONSULTING EDITOR

JÖRG MAYER, Dr. med. vet., M.Sc., DABVP (ECM), DECZM (small mammals), DACZM
Diplomate, American Board of Veterinary Practitioners (Exotic Companion Mammals); Diplomate, European College of Zoological Medicine (Small Mammals); Diplomate, American College of Zoological Medicine; Associate Professor of Zoological Medicine, Department of Small Animal Medicine and Surgery, University of Georgia College of Veterinary Medicine, Athens, Georgia, USA

EDITOR

SHANGZHE XIE, BSc/BVMS, MVS, PhD
Diplomate, American Board of Veterinary Practitioners (Avian Practice); Diplomate, Asian College of Conservation Medicine; Vice President, Veterinary Healthcare, Mandai Wildlife Group, Singapore

AUTHORS

ALI ANWAR BIN AHMAD, DVM (UPM), CertAqV
Diplomate for Asian College of Conservation Medicine; Veterinarian, Veterinary Healthcare, Mandai Wildlife Group, Singapore

PANAGIOTIS N. AZMANIS, DVM, PhD
Diplomate of European College of Zoological Medicine; Diplomate of Zoo and Wildlife Medicine (Royal College of Veterinary Surgeons); Dubai Falcon Hospital, Dubai, United Arab Emirates

HAMISH R. BARON, BVSc (Hons), PhD, FANZCVS (Avian Medicine and Surgery), MVetClinSci (Avian)
Veterinarian, The Unusual Pet Vets, Frankston, Victoria, Australia

DANIEL CALVO CARRASCO, LV, CertAVP(ZM), MRCVS
Diplomate, European College of Zoological Medicine (Avian); Assistant Vice President, Veterinary Healthcare, Mandai Wildlife Group, Singapore

IRINDI ÇITAKU, LMV
Veterinarian, Exotic Pets and Wildlife, Centro Veterinario México, Mexico City, Mexico

JOHANNES LODEWICUS COETZEE DE BEER, BVSc (Hons), MANZCVS (Avian Health)
Head of Service Centre for Avian, Reptiles and Exotics, Pellmeadow Estate, Klapmuts, South Africa

MARK MAGDY ERIAN, BVSc
Head of Exotic Animal Department of Rafiki Vet Hospital, Cairo, Egypt

JAMES HABERFIELD, BSc, BVMS, MANZCVS (Unusual Pets, Avian Medicine and Surgery)
Founder and Director, The Unusual Pet Vets, Frankston, Victoria, Australia

JEREMY Z.F. KAN, BVSc (Hons I)
Veterinarian, Concordia Pet Care, Happy Valley, Hong Kong

KATERINA C.L. LEUNG, BSc(Vet) (Hons I), BVSc (Hons I)
Veterinarian, Concordia Pet Care, Happy Valley, Hong Kong

QIANYING ATHENA LIM, BSc, BVMS
Exotic Companion Mammal Resident, Beecroft Animal Specialist & Emergency Hospital, Singapore

JI ZHEN LOW, BSc/BVMS, PGCert VetEd, FHEA
Manager, Diploma in Veterinary Technology, School of Applied Science, Temasek Polytechnic, Singapore

SEYED AHMAD MADANI, DVM, PhD
Assistant Professor, Department of Animal and Poultry Health and Nutrition, Faculty of Veterinary Medicine, University of Tehran, Tehran, Iran

RINA MAGUIRE, BVSc Hons1
Diplomate for American Board of Veterinary Practitioners - Exotic Companion Mammals; Diplomate for American College of Exotic Pet Medicine; Avian and Exotics, Beecroft Animal Specialist & Emergency Hospital, Singapore

NAQA SALEH MAHDI TAMIMI, DVM, PhD
Lecturer, Department of Internal and Preventive Medicine, College of Veterinary Medicine, University of Wasit, Wasit, Iraq

JORGE RIVERO, MVZ
Veterinarian, Sahuarita, Arizona, USA

AMIR ROSTAMI, DVM, PhD
Associate Professor, Department of Internal Medicine, Faculty of Veterinary Medicine, University of Tehran, Tehran, Iran

IZIDORA SLADAKOVIC, BVSc (Hons I), MVS
Diplomate of the American College of Zoological Medicine; Director, Avian & Exotics Service, Sydney, Australia

MOLLY VARGA SMITH, BVetMed DZooMed (Mammalian), MRCVS
Clinical Director Exotics Service, Rutland House Veterinary Referrals, Merseyside, United Kingdom

SHIWANI D. TANDEL, BVSc & AH, MVSc, MVetSci (Cons med)
Head Veterinarian, Exotic Animal Medicine, Phoenix Veterinary Specialty, Mumbai, India

CLAIRE VERGNEAU-GROSSET, DMV, IPSAV, CES
Diplomate of the American College of Zoological Medicine; Assistant Professor in Zoological Medicine, Faculty of Veterinary Medicine, Université de Montréal, Saint-Hyacinthe, Quebec, Canada

WEN-LIN WANG, DVM, MS
Veterinarian, Brave Vet Exotic Animal Veterinary Hospital, Taipei City, Taiwan

RYOTA WATANABE, DVM, BVSc, PhD, DÉS
Diplomate of the American College of Veterinary Anesthesia and Analgesia; Assistant
Professor in Anesthesia and Analgesia, Department of Small Animal Clinical Sciences,
School of Veterinary Medicine and Biomedical Sciences, Texas A&M University, College
Station, Texas, USA

SHANGZHE XIE, BSc/BVMS, MVS, PhD
Diplomate, American Board of Veterinary Practitioners (Avian Practice); Diplomate Asian
College of Conservation Medicine; Vice President, Veterinary Healthcare, Mandai Wildlife
Group, Singapore

ENRIQUE YARTO-JARAMILLO, DVM
Director, Exotic Pets and Wildlife, Centro Veterinario México, Mexico City, Mexico

Contents

> Laws regulating exotic animal ownership vary throughout the world. While some differences regarding the legal status and use of exotic companion animals are associated with cultural differences and public perception, some differences may result in different outcome, which could be of interest for other parts of the world. This article provides a general overview of relevant laws pertaining to exotic companion animals in certain developed countries.

> The diverse and unparalleled ecological landscape of Australasia has forged a unique environment for exotic animal practice, characterized by its rich biodiversity and stringent legislation. From its origins in the 1960s to its current status as a dedicated specialist niche, the exotic pet veterinary profession in Australasia has undergone a remarkable evolution. The profession faces hurdles in education and training, with limited dedicated institutes offering comprehensive programs, leading to a knowledge gap that employers must bridge. However, the close-knit community of passionate veterinarians has forged unique training pathways and opportunities, establishing a vibrant and highly skilled group of professionals.

> The objective of this clinical retrospective study was to analyze the prevalence and distribution of different avian and exotic animals presented to 2 exotics-only veterinary hospital in Hong Kong and Taiwan over a 1 year period. Exotic companion mammals, predominated by rabbits (*Oryctolagus cuniculus*) that were often diagnosed with fractures, were the most commonly presented group of patients in the hospital in Hong Kong while second most of that in Taiwan, with dental disease being commonly presented in the species. This study provided a general overview of avian and exotic patients presented to exotics-only practices in the East Asia region.

VETERINARY CLINICS OF NORTH AMERICA: EXOTIC ANIMAL PRACTICE

SERIES OF RELATED INTEREST

Veterinary Clinics: Small Animal Practice
https://www.vetsmall.theclinics.com/
Advances in Small Animal Care
https://www.advancesinsmallanimalcare.com

THE CLINICS ARE NOW AVAILABLE ONLINE!
Access your subscription at:
www.theclinics.com

Preface

No Man Is an Island

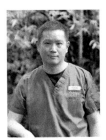

Shangzhe Xie, BSc/BVMS, MVS, PhD
Editor

The idea for this issue came about during a meeting of the international committee of the Association of Avian Veterinarians. The organization of these meetings was usually a complicated affair in itself, with the need to balance multiple time zones. The topic of the similarities and differences between one another's veterinary practices came up during this particular meeting and thus the seed for the issue was sown. The next step involved gathering authors from all around the world, some of whom did not previously know one another, to collaborate on articles relating to regions of the world. The format was left deliberately open so that there is flexibility to allow the unique aspects of each region to be showcased. The result was a diverse and eclectic mix of articles that truly reflects how wonderful it is to live in a world where nothing is the same, yet the common love for exotic animals connects a group of people with a common cause.

You will find articles that trace the history of the development of exotic animal practice in that part of the world. These articles pay homage to the pioneers of the field and the unique challenges of being the first to explore a field where the science was less developed than other aspects of veterinary medicine. Without these frontrunners who were willing to practice on the back of less than ideal scientific evidence, exotic animal practice would have never developed into the evidence-based frontier that it is today.

Other articles survey exotic animal practitioners around the region to identify their commonalities and difficulties. These articles highlight the human factors surrounding exotic animal practices. These human factors form a large part of how exotic animal practice evolves in each part of the world and are important to consider as the field continues to develop and move ahead. Some articles summarize the caseloads of exotic animal practices in different parts of the region that share a similar culture. These articles highlight the differences that can exist even within a region.

This is perhaps the least scientific issue of *Veterinary Clinics of North America: Exotic Animal Practice* in recent times, but it is important to take a moment to appreciate the

Vet Clin Exot Anim 27 (2024) xi–xii
https://doi.org/10.1016/j.cvex.2024.03.001

"art of veterinary science." It is also an important time to remember our similarities, rather than our differences, when there is so much international conflict going on around us. I, for one, am very grateful to be reminded of the international community that makes up exotic animal practice through the process of editing this issue, and that most importantly, no man is an island.

DISCLOSURE

There were no commercial or financial conflicts of interest and any funding sources to declare.

Shangzhe Xie, BSc/BVMS, MVS, PhD
Veterinary Healthcare
Mandai Wildlife Group
80 Mandai Lake Road
Singapore 729826

E-mail address:
shangzhe.xie@mandai.com

Legislative Differences Governing Exotic Animal Practice

Claire Vergneau-Grosset, DMV, IPSAV, CES, DACZM[a],*,
Ryota Watanabe, DVM, BVSc, PhD, DÉS, DACVAA[b],
Molly Varga Smith, BVetMed DZooMed (Mammalian), MRCVS[c],
Izidora Sladakovic, BVSc (Hons I), MVS, DACZM[d]

KEYWORDS

- Exotic pets • Laws • Ownership • Regulation

KEY POINTS

- State laws typically aim to protect native free-ranging animals from being kept as pets and restrict ownership of invasive species as pets, while importations and exportations of protected species are managed through the Convention on International Trade in Endangered Species of Wild Fauna and Flora.
- Depending on the state, different strategies are in place to prevent the release of exotic pets belonging to potentially invasive species. These strategies range from educating owners and delivering a permit, to completely prohibiting importation of such species and ownership as pets.
- State laws also aim to protect public health by avoiding introduction of zoonotic diseases when a country has a free status for a particular disease. For this reason, importation of certain species may be strongly regulated or prohibited. For instance, it is forbidden to import bats, raccoons, and prairie dogs to Japan.
- While numerous differences in regulations exist between countries, it is import to understand and respect these differences. Laws typically respond to evolving cultures and expectation of citizens regarding animal welfare. In addition, native species are in essence different among countries, and laws are created keeping in mind the protection of endemic and/or threatened species. While always perfectible, laws have led to variable results depending on the country of application. Comparing these results may help take a step back and think critically about our own regulations, as veterinarians may be involved as expert advisors in the process of law creation and revision.

[a] Université de Montréal, Saint-Hyacinthe, 3200 rue Sicotte, Saint-Hyacinthe, QC, J2S 2M2;
[b] Department of Small Animal Clinical Sciences, School of Veterinary Medicine and Biomedical Sciences, Texas A&M University, 660 Raymond Stotzer Parkingway, College Station, TX 77843, USA; [c] Rutland House Veterinary Referrals, Abbotsfield Road, St Helens, Merseyside, WA9 4HU;
[d] Avian & Exotics Service, 16 Myoora Road, Terrey Hills, New South Wales 2084, Australia
* Corresponding author. 3200 rue Sicotte, Saint-Hyacinthe, QC, J2S 2M2.
E-mail address: claire.grosset@umontreal.ca

Vet Clin Exot Anim 27 (2024) 465–487
https://doi.org/10.1016/j.cvex.2024.03.003
1094-9194/24/© 2024 Elsevier Inc. All rights reserved.
vetexotic.theclinics.com

INTRODUCTION

Keeping exotic animals as pets is a global practice. Although statistics are lacking in some countries, fish and birds are currently the third and the fourth most common companion pets in the United States, with 2.7% and 2.5% households owning a fish or a bird, respectively.[1] In Europe, companion birds are the third most common pets after dogs and cats,[2] while in Canada, fish are the most common pets.[3] With increasing numbers of zoologic companion animals, some citizens become increasingly aware of their welfare and associated challenges to keep them in urban environments.

In many developed countries, housing exotic pets is regulated through various legislative bodies. Legislation usually aims to address the challenges associated with exotic animal ownership, including limiting the risk of invasive species introduction, aiming to protect animal welfare, avoiding the escape of potentially dangerous animals, or limiting resistance to antibiotics, especially through drug residues contaminating water in aquatic species. While some differences in regulations are due to public perceptions and cultural differences, such as the prohibition of complete wing amputation in birds of prey or the special status of passerine bird Japanese white-eye (*Zosterops japonicus*) in Japan, outcomes obtained in certain areas of the world may serve as a source of inspiration for other countries.

This article aims to give an overview of the diverse regulations about exotic pet among countries around the globe. Of course, laws are in constant evolution. Thus, veterinary practitioners remain responsible for checking evolving legislations and discussing specific situations with their governmental agencies. This review article will not be a comprehensive summary but will rather highlight a few important points differing between exotic animal practice in North America and other countries worldwide, including Australia, Canada, the United Kingdom, countries of the European Union (EU), and Japan. All these countries are parties to the Convention on International Trade of Endangered Species. International regulations will not be covered here but the review will highlight differences among country regulations in regard to exotic animals. While regulations may be impacted by the geographic proximity of countries, historical factors may also play a role, such as the common history of countries in the Commonwealth, or the fact that Switzerland has remained outside of the EU and thus, has different laws.

OVERVIEW OF LAWS ABOUT EXOTIC ANIMALS IN THE COMMONWEALTH
Overview of Laws About Exotic Animals in Australia

Australia's delicate and unique ecosystem has had a significant impact on the legislation of exotic pet ownership. Deliberate and accidental introduction of pest species into Australia has caused major disturbances and destruction of this ecosystem through predation, competition with native wildlife for food, nests, and other resources, and introduction of diseases. Based on precedents and risk assessments of possible future introductions, laws currently prohibit many species being kept as pets in Australia, and importation and exportation of exotic pets is highly regulated.[4] Legislation is governed by both federal and state or territory wildlife authorities. General legislation will be discussed here, with some notable examples.

The abundance of native fauna in close proximity to people, particularly in the more populated states and cities (**Fig. 1**), means that many orphaned, injured, or diseased wildlife populations are rescued and taken into homes by well-meaning members of the public, who take it upon themselves to care for these animals. In some cases,

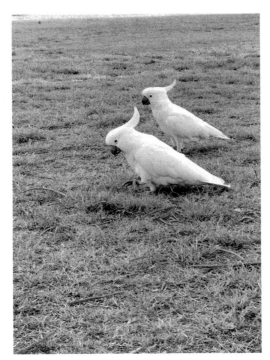

Fig. 1. Sulfur-crested cockatoos (*Cacatua galerita*) commonly flock in suburban areas.

these animals are kept as pets, and veterinary care may be sought some time later for these animals. It is generally not permitted to take protected native animals from the wild and keep them as pets. A permit may be sought for certain species in some states and territories. If a native animal is rescued by a person who is not a licensed rehabilitator, they must surrender the animal to a veterinarian or a licensed rehabilitator. Native animals can only stay under the care of licensed rehabilitators, and codes of practice dictate that these animals must be released into the wild once rehabilitated or, if rehabilitation and release are not possible, the animal should be euthanized.[5]

Native reptiles, such as bearded dragons (*Pogona vitticeps*), blue-tongued skinks (*Tiliqua scincoides*) and native pythons, and frogs can be kept as pets after obtaining the appropriate license from the state or territory authority. All pet reptiles and frogs need to have been bred in captivity. There are different license class levels depending on the species and number of animals to be kept. Reptiles covered by a basic license generally have basic husbandry requirements, whereas advanced license classes are required for more advanced and specialized species, including venomous reptiles. Some native species are not permitted in certain states and territories, whereas others may be exempt from a license. Owing to the high risk associated with deliberate or accidental release of non-native reptiles and amphibians into the wild, it is illegal to keep non-native reptiles as pets. Notable non-native reptiles that are illegal in Australia include red-eared sliders (*Trachemys scripta elegans*), boa constrictors (*Boa constrictor*), Burmese pythons (*Python bivittatus*), corn snakes (*Pantherophis guttatus*), chameleons (*Chamaeleonidae*), and leopard geckos (*Eublepharis macularius*).[6] The only non-native amphibian that can be kept without a license is the axolotl (*Ambystoma mexicanum*); however, axolotls are illegal in Northern Territory.

Reptile keepers must comply with the codes of practice within their state or territory, which cover the minimum husbandry standards required for the species. However, despite the availability of these resources, it is not uncommon for pet reptiles to present to exotics practitioners with common husbandry and dietary deficiencies, including calcium and ultraviolet B deficiency. The *Prevention of Cruelty to Animals Act 1979* prohibits the feeding of live vertebrate prey to reptiles.

Introduced carp (*Cyprinus carpio*) populations have become established in Australian waterways, disturbing the native environments and outnumbering the native fish. They are considered one of the most significant pest species in Australia and are only legal as pets in New South Wales, Western Australia, and the Australian Capital Territory, which has an impact on koi hobbyists.[7]

Many exotic mammals that are kept as pets around the world are illegal in Australia, such as chinchillas (*Chinchilla chinchilla*), hamsters (*Cricetidae*), and primates.[6] Exotic mammals that are permitted as pets are limited to rabbits (*Oryctolagus cuniculus*), guinea pigs (*Cavia porcellus*), ferrets (*Mustela putorius furo*), rats (*Rattus norvegicus*), and mice (*Mus musculus*), with some exceptions. Rabbits are one of the most commonly kept exotic pet mammals around the world and in Australia. Rabbits were introduced into Australia as a food source and for sport hunting but have become a pest with populations established and causing significant environmental and agricultural damage. While keeping rabbits as pets is permitted across most of Australia, they are illegal in Queensland.[8] Biologic control of pest rabbits using *Calicivirus* and *Myxoma* virus has put pet rabbits at risk and caused deaths of many pet rabbits.[9] The availability of vaccines to protect pet rabbits has been slow, with the vaccine against rabbit hemorrhagic disease virus 2 only becoming available in 2022. There is currently no vaccine against myxomatosis available in Australia. Keeping ferrets as pets is illegal in Queensland and Northern Territory. There are no established wild populations currently, however, as they are a predator species, introduction of ferrets into the wild has the potential to have disastrous consequences for Australian native fauna.[8]

Keeping native mammals is much more restricted compared to birds and reptiles. One of the major concerns with keeping native mammals as pets is their specialized husbandry requirements, which are difficult to provide, and natural biology of the species, making them unsuitable for captivity. Native mammal species are largely not permitted, with some species permitted with a license, depending on the state. Sugar gliders (*Petaurus breviceps*) are common as pets in North America, but are not permitted as pets across many parts of Australia. In some states, no native mammals are permitted as pets.[10]

Licensing requirements for native birds depend on the species but are generally least restrictive compared to other taxa. For example, for many commonly kept species, including budgerigars (*Melopsittacus undulatus*) and cockatiels (*Nymphicus hollandicus*), a license is not required. A license is required for some birds, with different license classes depending on the species. A license is not required for keeping of non-native birds in most states, and exotic psittacines commonly found in the pet trade around the world are similarly common in Australia. This is a welfare problem, particularly for long-lived psittacines that are relatively easy to acquire from pet shops and breeders. Some exotic psittacines are prohibited in some states, where introduction into the wild poses a high risk to the environment and agriculture. To prevent illegal pet trade of exotic birds, the government has implemented an exotic bird record-keeping scheme for breeders and bird keepers.[11] There are ongoing risk assessments of exotic psittacines, particularly regarding introduction of infectious diseases and the risk to the native psittacines. Keeping birds of prey as pets is illegal in Australia. Codes of practice are available from states and territories to ensure minimum husbandry requirements are provided to pet birds. However, similarly to reptiles, it is relatively common for pet birds to present to exotics practitioners with husbandry and dietary deficiencies.

Keeping of backyard poultry, particularly chickens, is increasingly common. In Australia, local councils set the rules and regulations on keeping of backyard poultry. Roosters are often prohibited in suburban areas. Medical treatment of poultry whose eggs are used for human consumption is a challenge as there are limited products that are licensed for use. Off-label use of products is permitted if a licensed product is not available, and the prescribing veterinarian is responsible for determining and recommending the appropriate withholding period.[12]

Pinioning of wings is not permitted and is considered an act of cruelty. Clipping of wing feathers of small birds and nervous birds is considered unacceptable in New South Wales.[13] In Victoria, wing clipping is only permitted under the guidance of a veterinarian experienced with birds and for the health of the individual bird.[14]

Codes of practice are available for keeping and sale of animals in pet shops, which include sections on exotic pets. Although these codes are in place to ensure that the basic requirements are provided and prospective owners are educated to protect the welfare of the animals, these are poorly enforced and it is up to the individual pet shop to ensure these guidelines are followed and the staff are trained and knowledgeable. Pet owners will often seek advice from pet shop staff and breeders, which may be incorrect. Policies to protect the welfare of exotic pets are still in their infancy, with policies and position statements available through the Australian Veterinary Association for small mammal dental guidelines, feeding of rabbits and guinea pigs, feeding of live mammals to snakes, and sale of unweaned altricial birds. The "Feeding of Rabbits and Guinea Pigs" policy states that these species must be fed a predominantly grass hay and/or grass diet and acknowledges the problems associated with muesli-type diets; however, the pet food industry is poorly regulated, and inappropriate foods are widely available and sold to misinformed pet owners.[15]

Despite the laws in place to protect the Australian environment and the welfare of exotic pets, there continues to be illegal smuggling, breeding, and keeping of species that are not permitted.[16] For legal exotic pets, guidelines are available to ensure that minimum requirements of these species are provided and their welfare protected. However, these guidelines are not sufficiently implemented, with owners commonly presenting their pets to exotics practitioners with husbandry-related illness. Ongoing refinement and policing of the guidelines are required to improve the welfare of exotic pets and protect the natural environment.

Overview of Laws About Exotic Animals in the United Kingdom

There are an estimated 42 million individual animals comprising more than 1000 species kept as pets in the United Kingdom.[17] Concerns surrounding the exotic pet trade contributing to species decline in the wild, its impact on ecosystems where individuals are caught directly from the wild, and stress/mortality of those individuals that are kept with poor husbandry all drive the discussion of how and indeed if certain species should be kept as pets. Within the United Kingdom, legislation applied to the keeping of exotic pets can be grouped into 3 categories: Public Health, Animal Welfare, and Wildlife/Habitat Protection.

The Dangerous Wild Animals Act 1976 relates to those species which cannot be kept in the United Kingdom without a specific license.[18] This legislation supports public safety and restricts the ownership of all animals considered dangerous to public health to individuals deemed fit to keep them safely. Potentially dangerous animals are included, for example all venomous species, crocodilians, and some ratites.

Licenses to keep those species covered under the Act are granted by the local government authority, and input of a suitably experienced veterinarian is often sought. This legislation does not affect a veterinarian's ability to treat these animals.

Hens and other waterfowl are increasingly being kept on a small scale in the United Kingdom, and often fall between being classed as food production animals and pet animals. Legally these animals are always viewed as potentially liable to become part of the human food chain (unlike horses, they cannot be exempted from this) and therefore must be kept and treated accordingly. For owners keeping poultry as pets, this can limit the variety of drugs that can legally be prescribed should that animal become unwell. Similar to the United States, there are some drugs that are prohibited for use in poultry (eg, chloramphenicol, metronidazole, ronidazole), while others have statutory egg (and meat) withdrawal times which the owner should be made aware of when the drugs are prescribed.[19] The challenge often comes when a pet hen is presented for a condition that is not infectious, but rather related to changes due to aging or traumatic damage. In these cases, the welfare of the animal remains paramount, and medications that support this can be prescribed as long as the veterinary surgeon makes detailed clinical notes regarding their reasoning and the owner is made aware of any potential risks should this bird enter the food chain.

The Welfare of Animals Act 2006/Welfare of Animals (Scotland) Act 2006 is the primary legislation governing the welfare of animals within the United Kingdom.[20] This Act not only makes it an offense to treat any captive animal cruelly (this includes captive wildlife) but also an offense to omit or do something that will cause an animal to suffer at some time in the future. Within the remit of this Act are both physical acts (prohibited surgical procedures deemed mutilations, including but not limited to scent gland removal in ferrets, pinioning of wings in waterfowl over 10 days of age without an anesthetic) and husbandry deficits. All animals in captivity must have a suitable environment, a suitable diet, the ability to exhibit normal behaviors, housing with or without other animals as appropriate for the species and protection from pain suffering, injury, and disease. This puts the onus on the keeper of an exotic species to research and provide suitable care for that animal.

The Wildlife and Countryside Act 1981 and its amendments offer protection to wild species in the United Kingdom,[21] making it an offense to take, injure or kill a protected species, disturb a protected species in its nest or shelter, possess a protected species, release or allow to escape into the wild any nonindigenous species (such as Eastern gray squirrels [*Sciurus carolinensis*], Canada geese [*Branta canadensis*], and sika deer [*Cervus nippon*] that have established wild populations in the United Kingdom but are not native species; **Fig. 2**) or species listed in Schedule 9 of the Act (including animals that are no longer established in the wild in the United Kingdom such as wild boar [*Sus scrofa*]). This act limits the species that may be kept in captivity legally within the United Kingdom and discourages the keeping of wild animals that are not fit for release, in long-term captivity, unless there is a specific conservation need.

Overview of Laws About Exotic Animals in Canada

In Canada, provincial or federal regulations apply depending on the classification of the species. Migratory birds except birds of prey, marine mammals, and marine fish are under federal jurisdiction. Other birds, terrestrial mammals, and freshwater fish are under provincial jurisdiction. The laws of the province of Quebec will be presented as an example. Since 2018, laws regarding the possession of nondomestic animals have been updated in Quebec to include specific husbandry requirements.[22] For instance, it is forbidden to hand raise an exotic cat unless a medical condition precludes natural feeding by its mother. Shade and an appropriate temperature gradient

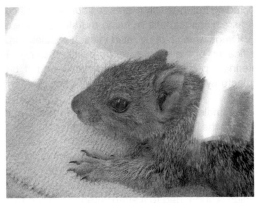

Fig. 2. An orphaned Eastern gray squirrel (*Sciurus carolinensis*) rehabilitated in the United Kingdom must not be released into the wild based on the Wildlife and Countryside Act.

should be available at all time for all animals. The listed zoonotic pathogens should be screened for on necropsies.[22] This law does not apply to rabbits, pot-bellied pigs, ferrets, guinea pigs, or pigeons, which are considered domestic species in Quebec.[23] These species are protected by the Animal Welfare and Safety Act, which defines abuse and requires any veterinarian to report any case of abuse to the authorities.[23] A professional permit is mandatory to own certain nondomestic species, such as servals (*Leptailurus serval*), kangaroos (*Macropus* spp), or Burmese pythons.[24] Individuals applying for a permit must document a 1 to 3 year experience taking care of a related species depending on the class of permit. The permit, which is renewable yearly, is conditioned to the signature of licensed veterinarian in Quebec, who is responsible for the welfare of the animals of the collection. In addition, certain conditions apply to own dangerous animals, for example, anybody acquiring a venomous reptile should have liability insurance covering 2 million dollars of damages,[24] which has a dissuasive effect.

While many laws regarding veterinary practice are very similar to laws in the United States, some differences exist. Some drugs may be approved for exotic animals in the United States but not in Canada (this is the case for some antiparasitic treatments containing selamectin or deslorelin implants). In birds of prey, when a bird is nonreleasable and should undergo a wing amputation for medical reasons, there is no limitation regarding the way amputations should be performed. A recent retrospective study including captive birds amputated proximal to the shoulder showed that their life expectancy was higher than that of other rehabilitated birds of prey kept in captivity. Few complications were associated with the wing stump, suggesting that this practice may be appropriate if patients are carefully selected.[25]

OVERVIEW OF LAWS ABOUT EXOTIC ANIMALS IN THE EUROPEAN UNION

In the EU, legislation regarding exotic and food animals is made by the European Commission and translated into legislation in each member state (country), which can be more restrictive. In the EU, rabbits are considered minor food animal species,[26] although companion rabbit breeds are listed as domestic in some countries.[27] Pigs and chicken considered major food animal species, including companion pot-bellied pigs and backyard chickens. Salmons (*Salmo* spp) are considered major food-producing species in the EU, while other fish are classified as minor food-producing species.[26] In some EU countries, several ornamental fish species are considered domestic animals, including koi, goldfish (*Carassius auratus*), and certain mutations of exotic animals, such as albinos axolotls or lutino mutations of Alexandrine parakeets (*Psittacula eupatria*).[27] Drugs which can be used in each species, especially antibiotics, depend on the classification of the species as domestic, major, or minor food animal species. Certain veterinary procedures performed are banned on ethical grounds, including ferret sacculectomy (ie, scent gland removal) when performed for nonmedical reasons.[28]

Ownership of exotic animals is regulated at the level of the EU, and states' laws may be more restrictive than at the European level. For instance, in France, venomous reptiles, snakes and monitor lizards measuring more than 3 m as adults, crocodilians, carnivores weighing more than 6 kg, mygalomorphae, and among others are classified as dangerous animals.[29] Anyone willing to acquire a dangerous animal legally needs to go through a training of about 2 weeks about the species acquired, to write a thesis about the species, which is submitted to a state veterinarian and to present its request to the regional authorities. This gives them a certification of ability allowing to own the species under certain conditions (**Fig. 3**). The same process is applied to individuals acquiring fragile species or breeding birds, reptiles, or certain exotic mammals above a certain number of individuals. A certification of ability is required to own a lemur, for instance, or a chameleon except for panther (*Furcifer pardalis*) or veiled chameleons (*Chamaeleo calyptratus*).[30]

Importation of certain species to Europe may be prohibited to prevent entry of foreign animal diseases. In particular, importation of pet birds has been prohibited for a few years to prevent introduction of avian influenza. Ironically, avian influenza is currently endemic in Europe and it is thought that natural bird migrations were the source of introduction of the current avian influenza strain.[31]

Similar to the extra-label drug use in the United States, extra-label drug use is possible for veterinarians treating minor species under certain conditions.[26] Regarding the use of medications in food animal species, withdrawal times are based on the maximal residue levels defined by the European Food Safety Authority. Prohibited drugs for food animal species are listed in Annex IV of the European Regulations and include chloramphenicol, chlorpromazine, colchicine, dimetridazole, metronidazole, nitrofurans, and ronidazole (European Union CEE 2377/1990), which is a list very similar to the one found in the United States. Some EU countries further prohibit the use of certain antibiotics in all animal species, which may include vancomycin,

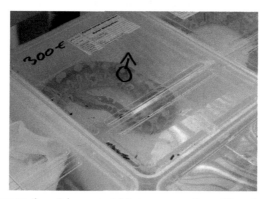

Fig. 3. Acquiring more than 3 boa constrictors or more than 40 snakes of any species is forbidden without a certification of ability delivered by local authorities in France (Picture from the Hamm Terraristika reptile show, Germany).

certain fluoroquinolones, third- and fourth-generation cephalosporins such as ceftazidime, and antibiotics used against mycobacteriosis. In addition, certain antibiotics, such as enrofloxacin, can only be used after a bacterial culture has determined that bacteria are susceptible exclusively to this antibiotic.[32]

OVERVIEW OF LAWS ABOUT EXOTIC ANIMALS IN ASIA, EXAMPLE OF JAPAN

In Japan, the species targeted by veterinary medicine began with large animals such as horses and cows and expanded over time to companion animals such as dogs and cats, as well as laboratory animals such as mice and rats.[33] As a result of environmental pollution during the period of rapid economic growth after World War II, environmental issues became increasingly serious in the 1970s and 1980s. This led to a decrease in wild animals, raising awareness of the need for their protection. Consequently, new zoos and aquariums were established, and wildlife protection centers were set up in various locations. Furthermore, the pet boom in Japan led to the importation of wild animals from around the world, and they were kept in large numbers as so-called exotic pets. Owing to this societal background, the importance of medical care and research for wild animals increased, gradually leading to the inclusion of wild animals as a focus in the field of veterinary medicine. It is said that there are over 4000 species of wild mammals worldwide, and approximately 130 species inhabit Japan, with over 30% being endemic species.[34] Despite its small land area, Japan has a variety of endemic mammalian species due to being isolated from the continent since the glacial period. This includes numerous endemic species such as rodents and bats. Additionally, it is estimated that over 9000 island species exist in the world, among which 542 species inhabit Japan.[35] Keeping free-ranging animals as pets was previously somewhat accepted, but the capture and keeping of such animals for companionship have been restricted since 1950. Since 2007, only one species, the passerine bird Japanese white-eye, which is native from Japan and was traditionally used for song contests, is allowed to be captured and kept for companionship per household.[36] Subsequently, in the 2011 revision of the guidelines, capturing free-ranging animals for companionship is usually not permitted.[36]

In Japan, veterinary medicine is under the jurisdiction of the Ministry of Agriculture, Forestry and Fisheries, which also oversees animal pharmaceuticals. The Veterinary Surgeons Act established by the Ministry of Agriculture, Forestry and Fisheries recognizes "the medical treatment of kept animals" as an exclusive task of veterinarians. The specified animals for medical treatment include horses, domestic sheep, wild sheep, pigs, dogs, cats, chickens, quails, all species of the Psittacidae family, all species of the Estrildidae family, and all species of the thrush (Turdidae) family.[37] The laws regarding the use of medications for exotic animals are fundamentally similar to those for other companion animals. Certain drugs are prohibited for food animal species. However, there are exceptions, such as when a veterinarian uses them for diagnosis, treatment, or prevention of diseases related to the subject of their medical care.[38] Thus, prescribing enrofloxacin in a pet chicken in a context of treatment would be legal for veterinarians in Japan.

The Welfare and Management of Animals Act[39] protects domestic rabbits, chickens, domestic ducks, and domestic pigeons among exotic pets. Additionally, other animals kept by humans, belonging to the mammalian, avian or reptilian classes, are also subject to the law, but not free-ranging animals of the same species, fish, or invertebrates.[40] Offenses under this act include (1) injuring these animals, (2) maliciously withholding feed or water, overworking, or restraining them in a place where maintaining their health and safety is difficult, (3) failing to provide proper protection if the cared-for animals become sick or injured, (4) keeping animals in facilities where excrement has accumulated or in facilities where the corpses of other cared-for animals are left unattended, (5) any other forms of abuse, and (6) abandoning cared-for animals. Offenders of these provisions are subject to penalties under the law.

As mentioned earlier, Japan has numerous endemic species. However, for academic, educational purposes, and due to recent trends such as the exotic animal boom, there are cases where animals are imported from overseas. Being an island nation, Japan places great importance on preventing the introduction of infectious diseases from other continents and the destruction of ecosystems. Therefore, various quarantine systems have been established to safeguard against these risks.

Rabies Prevention Act

Japan is one of the few countries in the world with no incidence of rabies, and as a result, its export–import quarantine measures are strictly regulated.[41] Under the Rabies Prevention Act, animals subject to quarantine include not only dogs and cats but also raccoons, foxes, and skunks. Additionally, the import of bats has been prohibited since 2003.

Exotic Animal Importation

Laws regarding exotic animal importation in Japan are based on risk assessment for foreign diseases importation and introduction of invasive species to the wild. Importation of exotic animals mandates notification to the Ministry of Health, Labor and Welfare, which is in charge of human health.[42] This system aims to prevent the introduction of zoonotic diseases by ensuring appropriate hygiene management in the exporting country. The system applies to land mammals, excluding prohibited species (**Table 1**) and regulates quarantined animals (artiodactyls, chickens, quails, ostriches, partridges, turkeys, ducks, and geese, rabbits, and bees). Quarantined animals include rodents (hamsters, squirrels, guinea pigs, and chinchillas), lagomorphs,

Table 1 List of import-prohibited animals in Japan		
Disease to be Prevented	**Animals**	**Prohibited Area**
Ebola, Marburg	Monkey	All areas For testing and research or for display (to be kept at testing and research institutes or zoos), approved only from the United States, Indonesia, Guyana, Cambodia, Suriname, China, Philippines, and Vietnam. (Monkeys from other regions and monkeys that have passed through other regions are not imported.)
Plague Severe acute respiratory syndrome Nipah virus infection and lyssavirus infection. Lassa fever	Prairie dog Weasel badgers, raccoons, civets Bat Soft-furred rats	All areas

Japanese Animal Quarantine Service Web site.[35] The Ornithological Society Of Japan *Check list of Japanese Birds* 2012. *Adapted from* The Ornithological Society Of Japan Check list of Japanese Birds 2012. Available from: https://ornithology.jp/katsudo/Publications/Checklist7_e.html, Accessed January 9th 2024.

Table 2
List of Regulated Living Organisms under the Invasive Alien Species Act in Japan (excerpted only mammals, birds, reptiles, amphibians, and fish)

Class	Order	Family	Genus	Invasive Alien Species
Mammalia	Marsupialia	Phalangeridae	Trichosurus	Brushtail possum (T vulpecula)
	Insectivora	Erinaceidae	Erinaceus	Any species of the genus Erinaceus
	Primates	Cercopithecidae	Macaca	Taiwan macaque (M cyclopis)
				Crab-eating macaque (M fascicularis)
				Rhesus macaque (M mulatta)
				Taiwan macaque × Japanese macaque (M cyclopis × M fuscata)
				Rhesus macaque × Japanese macaque (M mulatta × M fuscata)
	Rodentia	Myocastoridae	Myocastor	Coypu or nutria (M coypus)
		Sciuridae	Callosciurus	Pallas's squirrel or Taiwan squirrel (C erythraeus)
				Finlayson's squirrel (C finlaysonii)
			Pteromys	Russian (or Siberian) flying squirrel (P volans) excluding Japanese subspecies (P volans orii)
			Sciurus	Gray squirrel (S carolinensis)
				Eurasian red squirrel (S vulgaris) excluding Japanese subspecies (S vulgaris orientis)
		Muridae	Ondatra	Muskrat (O zibethicus)
		Procyonidae	Procyon	Crab-eating raccoon (P cancrivorus)
				Raccoon (P lotor)
	Carnivora	Mustelidae	Mustela	American mink (M vison)
		Herpestidae	Herpestes	Small Indian mongoose (H auropunctatus)
				Javan mongoose (H javanicus)
			Mungos	Banded mongoose (M mungo)
	Artiodactyla	Cervidae	Axis	All species of the genus Axis
			Cervus	All species of the genus Cervus excluding C nippon centralis, C nippon keramae, C nippon mageshimae, C nippon nippon, C nippon pulchellus, C nippon yakushimae, C nippon yesoensis
			Dama	All species of the genus Dama
			Elaphurus	Pere David's deer (E davidianus)
			Muntiacus	Reeves's muntjac (M reevesi)

(continued on next page)

Table 2
(continued)

Class	Order	Family	Genus	Invasive Alien Species
Aves	Anseriformes	Anatidae	Branta	Canada goose (B canadensis)
	Passeriformes	Pycnonotidae	Pycnonotus	Red-vented bulbul (P cafer)
		Timaliidae	Garrulax	Laughing thrushes (Gcanorus)
				Moustached laughingthrush (G cineraceus)
				Masked laughingthrush (G perspicillatus)
				White-browed laughingthrush (G sannio)
			Leiothrix	Red-billed mesia (L lutea)
Reptilia	Testudinata	Chelydridae	Chelydra	Snapping turtle (C serpentina)
		Emydidae	Trachemys	Common slider (T scripta)
		Geoemydidae	Mauremys	M sinensis
				M sinensis × M japonica
				M sinensis × M mutica
				M sinensis × M reevesii
	Squamata	Agamidae	Japalura	J swinhonis
		Iguanidae (Polychrotidae)	Anolis	Bueycito anole (A allogus)
				Blue-eyed grass-bush anole, Monte Verde anole (A alutaceus)
				Twig anole (A angusticeps)
				Green anole (A carolinensis)
				Knight anole (A equestris)
				Garman anole (A garmanni)
				Habana anole, Cuban white-fanned anole (A homolechis)
				Brown anole (A sagrei)
		Colubridae	Boiga	Green cat snake (B cyanea)
				Dog-toothed cat snake (B cynodon)
				Gold-ringed cat snake, Mangrove snake (B dendrophila)
				Brown tree snake (B irregularis)
				Black-headed cat snake (B nigriceps)
		Viperidae	Elaphe	Taiwan beauty snake (E taeniura friesi)
			Protobothrops	Taiwan pit vipers (P mucrosquamatus)

Class	Order	Family	Genus	Common name (species)
Amphibia	Anura	Bufonidae	Bufo	Great plains toad (B cognatus) Spotted toad (B guttatus) Cane toad (B marinus) B melanostictus Red-spotted toad (B punctatus) Oak toad (B quercicus) Texas toad (B speciosus) South American common toad (B typhonius)
		Hylidae	Osteopilus	Cuban tree frog (O septentrionalis)
		Leptodactylidae	Eleutherodactylus	Puerto Rican coqui (E coqui) E johnstonei Greenhouse frog (E planirostris)
		Microhylidae	Kaloula	K pulchra
		Ranidae	Rana	Bullfrog (R catesbeiana)
		Rhacorhoridae	Polypedates	Asian tree frog (P leucomystax)
Osteichthyes	Lepisosteiformes	Lepisosteidae	Atractosteus Lepisosteus	Any member of the family Lepisosteidae Any living hybrid organisms of species of the family Lepisosteidae
	Cypriniformes	Cyprinidae	Acheilognathus	A macropterus
	Siluriformes	Bagridae	Tachysurus	T fulvidraco
		Ictaluridae	Ameiurus	A nebulosus
			Ictalurus	Channel catfish (I punctatus)
			Pylodictis	P olivaris
		Siluridae	Silurus	S glanis
	Esociformes	Esocidae	Esox	Any species of the family Esocidae Any living hybrid organisms of species of family Esocidae
	Cyprinodontiformes	Poeciliidae	Gambusia	Western mosquito fish (G affinis) G holbrooki

(continued on next page)

Table 2
(continued)

Class	Order	Family	Genus	Invasive Alien Species
	Perciformes (Percoidei)	Centrarchidae	Lepomis	Bluegill (*L macrochirus*)
			Micropterus	Smallmouth bass (*M dolomieu*)
				Largemouth bass (*M salmoides*)
		Gobiidae	Neogobius	N melanostomus
		Centropomidae	Lates	L niloticus
			Morone	M americana
				White bass (*M chrysops*)
				Striped bass (*M saxatilis*)
				Striped bass × white bass (*M chrysops* × *M saxatilis*)
		Percidae	Gymnocephalus	G cernuus
			Perca	Eurasian perch (*P fluviatilis*)
			Sander (*Stizostedion*)	Pikeperch (*S lucioperca*)
		Sinipercidae	Siniperca	Mandarin fish (*S chuatsi*)
				Golden mandarin fish (*S scherzeri*)

Adapted from[44] Japanese Ministry of the Environment Web site *List of Regulated Living Organisms under the Invasive Alien Species Act in Japan* 2020. Available at: https://www.env.go.jp/nature/intro/2outline/list.html, Accessed January 9 2024.

Table 3
Examples of mammals whose ownership is regulated in each region, restriction applied, and main rationale associated with each regulation

	Australia	Canada	United Kingdom	Europe	Japan
Exotic species	Rabbits, ferrets, guinea pigs, rats, mice	Large Felidae, nonhuman primates, dromedaries	Eastern gray squirrels, boars	All marsupials including sugar glider and hedgehogs	1. Chiroptera, prairie dogs, raccoons, weasel badgers, primates 2. Squirrels, hedgehogs, mongoose
Restriction applied	Only species allowed (except rabbits and ferrets in Queensland and ferrets in Northern Territory; some native mammals are permitted only in some areas)	Require a permit (signed by a veterinarian responsible of their welfare)	Ownership discouraged and release is an offense	Require a permit (thesis and oral evaluation by the authorities)	Prohibited
Rationale	Risk of invasive species to the local fauna	Risk to the public and animal welfare	Risk of invasive species to the local fauna	Animal welfare	1. Biosafety 2. Risk of invasive species to the local fauna

Table 4
Examples of reptiles and amphibians whose ownership is regulated in each region, restriction applied, and main rationale associated with each regulation

	Australia	Canada	United Kingdom	Europe	Japan
Reptile groups	Any non-native species except axolotl	1. Venomous species, large snakes (>2.4 m), crocodilians and monitor lizards >0.9 m) (in some provinces) 2. Native species (eg, wood turtles)	Venomous species, crocodilians	1. Venomous species, large snakes, crocodilians, monitor lizards >4 m 2. Native species (eg, rainbow boa in French Guyana) 3. Fragile species such as Trionychidae	Red-eared slider, snapping turtles, anoles, Bufo toads
Restriction applied	License required	1. License and insurance required 2. Permit required (signed by a veterinarian responsible of their welfare)	License required	License required	Prohibited
Rationale	Risk of invasive species to the local fauna	Risk to the public and wild animals protection	Risk to the public	Risk to the public and wild animals protection	Risk of invasive species to the local fauna

Table 5
Examples of birds whose ownership is regulated in each region, restriction applied, and main rationale associated with each regulation

	Australia	Canada	United Kingdom	Europe	Japan
Avian groups	Some native and exotic psittacines	Most birds of prey	Canada geese	Ramphastidae, many birds of prey (in some countries)	Canada geese
Restriction applied	License required in some states	License required	Prohibited	License required	Prohibited
Rationale	Risk of invasive species to the local fauna	Animal welfare, protection of free-ranging species	Risk of invasive species to the local fauna	Animal welfare, protection of free-ranging species	Risk of invasive species to the local fauna

Table 6
Examples of fish whose ownership is regulated in each region, restriction applied, and main rationale associated with each regulation

	Australia	Canada	United Kingdom	Europe	Japan
Fish groups	Koi carp	Copper redhorse	Large mouthed black bass	Lionfish	Striped bass, Eurasian perch, Lepisosteidae, channel catfish, smallmouth bass, largemouth bass
Restriction applied	Prohibited except in New South Wales, Western Australia, and the Australian Capital Territory	License required (endangered endemic fish species)	Release prohibited	License required	Prohibited
Rationale	Risk of invasive species to the local fauna	Animal welfare, protection of free-ranging species	Risk of invasive species to the local fauna	Risk to the public	Risk of invasive species to the local fauna

other land mammals (ferrets, wallabies, sugar gliders, hedgehogs [*Erinaceus* spp and *Atelerix* spp]), and birds (psittacine birds, buntings [old world passerines], and pigeons). Confirmation of proper hygiene management in the exporting country is required to prevent the entry of zoonotic diseases. When importing these targeted animals, it is necessary to submit documents to the Ministry of Health, Labor and Welfare quarantine office, including a health certificate issued by the exporting country's government agency and a declaration form specifying the type and quantity of animals. It is important to note that this system applies not only to animals imported for sale or exhibition but also to companion animals kept by individuals. For rodents such as hamsters, guinea pigs, many species of squirrels, and chinchillas, stringent import conditions are in place due to their potential as sources of zoonotic infections. For animals kept at home overseas or purchased from pet shops abroad, it is often challenging to meet these requirements, making it generally impossible to bring them back to Japan.

Act on the Prevention of Adverse Ecological Impacts Caused by Designated Specific Invasive Alien Species

"Specific alien species" refers to alien species (species of foreign origin, including those resulting from hybridization; **Table 2**) that are individually designated by a Cabinet Order as capable of causing harm to ecosystems, human life and body, agriculture, forestry, and fisheries.[43] Under this act, the breeding and keeping of specific alien species are prohibited. Individuals intending to breed or keep specific alien species for purposes such as academic research or other purposes specified in ministerial ordinances must obtain permission from the competent minister. When granted permission for breeding, measures must be taken. These include regularly confirming the situation of breeding, conducting maintenance inspections of facilities, and taking measures such as placing microchips, tags or leg bands, and displaying signs or photographs to make clear that permission has been granted for breeding of the specific alien species. Importation, breeding, sale, transfer, and other movements including release are prohibited except for those individuals who have obtained permission. Specific alien species must not be transferred, given, delivered, and received (including sales).

SUMMARY

In summary, many differences in state laws may be noted (**Tables 3–6**). However, the general principles regarding exotic animal ownership regulation are similar in all cited countries. Animal welfare and conservation is one of these principles. Concerns surrounding the exotic pet trade contributing to species decline in the wild, its impact on ecosystems where individuals are caught directly from the wild, and stress/mortality of those individuals that are transported or kept with poor husbandry all drive the discussion of how and indeed if certain species should be kept as pets. Another principle is public health and safety. With this goal in mind, importation of certain species that are potential reservoirs of rabies, plague, avian influenza, or other zoonotic disease is prohibited in certain countries that are free of these diseases. Dangerous animal ownership is also regulated in various ways depending on the country, which range from complete prohibition to obligation to have an insurance in case this animal was to harm another citizen. A general goal is the prevention of introduction of invasive species to the wild, justifying the prohibition of chinchillas, hamsters, birds of prey, and non-native reptile and amphibian species as pets in Australia, or red-eared sliders in Japan, similar to the prohibition to hedgehogs and ferrets in California. Depending on the culture, prohibiting the keeping of certain exotic species may be more or less accepted. Other barriers, such as penalties, are implemented in other countries to prevent the release of pets of invasive species. Finally, some veterinary procedures performed in North America may be prohibited in certain countries, such as ferret scent gland excision or bird pinioning. On the contrary, certain procedures forbidden in the United States such as amputation of captive birds proximal to the elbow are allowed in other countries. Evaluating the outcome of these various policies may help improve regulations regarding exotic animals and ultimately their care.

CLINICS CARE POINTS

- It is illegal to keep chinchillas, hamsters, birds of prey, and non-native reptile and amphibian species in Australia, except for axolotls in some areas.
- It is illegal to import certain species in Japan, such as prairie dogs, raccoons, and all bat species. It is also forbidden to keep or breed potentially invasive species in Japan, including cane toads, snapping turtles, red-eared sliders, channel catfish, or Canada geese.
- Keeping as pets certain nondomestic species, such as servals, nondomestic primates, birds of prey, or large reptiles, requires a permit in Quebec.
- Exotic pet owners and breeders must demonstrate their abilities through a written thesis and take an oral test, to keep more than a certain number of exotic animals in some European countries (>25 leopard geckos for instance).
- Some procedures historically performed in zoologic companion animals are forbidden in certain countries, including pinioning of birds in Australia and routine scent gland excision in ferrets in Europe and in the United Kingdom.

DISCLOSURE

The authors have nothing to disclose.

REFERENCES

1. American Veterinary Medical Association. Pet ownership and demographics Sourcebook. 2022. Available at: https://ebusiness.avma.org/files/Product Downloads/eco-pet-demographic-report-22-low-res.pdf. [Accessed 9 January 2024].
2. Bedford E. Pet population in Europe 2022, by animal type. 2022. Available at: https://www.statista.com/statistics/453880/pet-population-europe-by-animal/. [Accessed 9 January 2024].
3. Bedford E. Total pet population in Canada 2020, by type. 2020. Available at: https://www.statista.com/statistics/1255033/pet-population-by-type-canada/. [Accessed 9 January 2024].
4. Henderson W, Bomford M. Detecting and preventing incursions of exotic animals in Australia, . Invasive animals Cooperative research centre canberra.
5. New South Whale Government Office of Environment & Heritage. Code of practice for injured, sick and orphaned protected fauna 2011.
6. Toomes A, Stringham OC, Mitchell L, et al. Australia's wish list of exotic pets: biosecurity and conservation implications of desired alien and illegal pet species. NeoBiota 2020;60:43–59.
7. Australian Government - the Fisheries Research and Development Corporation. The National Carp Control Plan. 2022. Available at: https://www.agriculture.gov.

au/biosecurity-trade/pests-diseases-weeds/pest-animals-and-weeds/national-carp-control-plan#:~:text=The%20NCCP%20is%20the%20largest,and%20over%2040%20research%20scientists. [Accessed 9 January 2024].

8. Queensland Government Pets you can't keep in Queensland. 2022. Available at: https://www.daf.qld.gov.au/__data/assets/pdf_file/0011/1629596/pets-you-cant-keep-in-qld.pdf. [Accessed January 9, 2024].
9. Invasive Plants and Animals Committee. Australian pest animal strategy 2017 to 2027. Canberra: Australian Government Department of Agriculture and Water Resources; 2016. p. 56.
10. Cooney R, Chapple R, Doornbos S, et al. Australian Native Mammals as Pets: a feasibility study into conservation, welfare and industry aspects. Canberra: Australian Government Rural Industries Research and Development Corporation; 2010.
11. Australian Government - Department of the Environment And Energy. Compliance and record keeping guide for ownership of exotic birds in Australia 2018. p. 16.
12. Gray P, Jenner R, Norris J, et al, Ltd Australian Veterinary Association, and Australia Animal Medicines. Antimicrobial prescribing guidelines for poultry. Aust Vet J 2021;99(6):181–235.
13. Nsw Government Department of. Primary Industries NSW Code of Practice No 4 - Keeping and Trading of Birds.
14. Environment and Climate Action Department of Energy *Code of Practice for the Housing of Caged Birds, Animal Welfare Victoria*. 2023. Available at: https://agriculture.vic.gov.au/livestock-and-animals/animal-welfare-victoria/domestic-animals-act/codes-of-practice/code-of-practice-for-the-housing-of-caged-birds. [Accessed 9 January 2024].
15. Australian Veterinary Association *Policies and Position Statements: Feeding rabbits and guinea pigs*. 2015. Available at: https://www.ava.com.au/policy-advocacy/policies/unusual-pets-and-avian/feeding-rabbits-and-guinea-pigs/. [Accessed 9 January 2024].
16. Toomes Adam, García-Díaz Pablo, Wittmann Talia A, et al. New aliens in Australia: 18 years of vertebrate interceptions. Wildl Res 2020;47(1):55–67.
17. Burke M, Sutherland N, Ares E. In: Library 0124 HoC, editor. Exotics pets trade debate pack CDP 2015. 2015.
18. Uk Public General Act *Dangerous Wild Animals Act* 1976. Available at: www.legislation.gov.uk. [Accessed 9 January 2024].
19. Polland G. Legal Issues. In: Polland G, editor. BSAVA manual of backyard poultry medicine and surgery. Gloucester, UK: BSAVA; 2019.
20. Available at:UK public general acts *animal welfare act* www.legislation.gov.uk. [Accessed 9 January 2024].
21. UK public general acts *Wildlife and Countryside act*. . [Accessed 9 January 2024].
22. Available at:Ministère De La Faune Des Forêts Et Des Parcs *Loi sur la conservation et la mise en valeur de la faune* https://www.legisquebec.gouv.qc.ca/fr/document/rc/C-61.1,%20r.%205.1. [Accessed 9 January 2024].
23. Parliament Of Quebec *Animal welfare and safety act*. 2023. Available at: https://www.legisquebec.gouv.qc.ca/en/document/cs/B-3.1. [Accessed 9 January 2024].
24. Ministère De La Faune Des Forêts Et Des Parcs *Règlement sur les permis de garde d'animaux en captivité*. 2018. Available at: https://www.legisquebec.gouv.qc.ca/fr/document/rc/C-61.1,%20r.%2020.1.1/. [Accessed 9 January 2024].

25. Aymen J, Fitzgerald G, Lair S, et al. Outcomes of birds of prey with surgical or traumatic wing amputation: a retrospective study from 1995 to 2017. J Avian Med Surg 2022;36(1):14–20.

26. The European Agency for the Evaluation of Medicinal Products *Points to consider regarding efficacy requirements for minor species and minor indications*. Available at: Vet Med Int 2002;16 http://www.ema.europa.eu/docs/en_GB/document_library/Scientific_guideline/2009/10/WC500004682.pdf. [Accessed 9 January 2024].

27. Ministère De L'Écologie Et Du Développement Durable *Arrêté du 11 août 2006 fixant la liste des espèces, races ou variétés d'animaux domestiques*. Available at: Journal Officiel de la République Française 2006;5 https://www.legifrance.gouv.fr/affichTexte.do?cidTexte=JORFTEXT000000789087&dateTexte=&categorieLien=id. [Accessed 9 January 2024].

28. Jekl V, Casales S. Soft tissue surgery: ferrets. In: Quesenberry K, et al, editors. Ferrets, rabbits, and rodents clinical medicine and surgery. Saint Louis, MO: Elsevier; 2021. p. 432–45.

29. Ministère De L'aménagement Du Territoire Et De L'environnement *Arrêté du 21 novembre 1997 définissant deux catégories d'établissements, autres que les établissements d'élevage, de vente et de transit des espèces de gibier dont la chasse est autorisée, détenant des animaux d'espèces non domestiques*. Available at: Journal Officiel de la République Française 2017; https://www.legifrance.gouv.fr/loda/id/LEGIARTI000034369738/2017-04-06/. [Accessed 9 January 2024].

30. Ministère De La Transition Écologique Et Solidaire *Arrêté du 8 octobre 2018 fixant les règles générales de détention d'animaux d'espèces non domestiques*. Available at: Journal Officiel de la République Française 2018; https://www.legifrance.gouv.fr/loda/id/LEGIARTI000037495937/2018-10-14/. [Accessed 9 January 2024].

31. European Centre for Disease Prevention And Control *Avian influenza overview April – June 2023*. 2023. Available at: https://www.ecdc.europa.eu/sites/default/files/documents/AI-Report%20XXV_final.pdf. [Accessed 9 January 2024].

32. Ministère De L'agriculture De L'agroalimentaire Et De La Forêt *Arrêté du 18 mars 2016 fixant la liste des substances antibiotiques d'importance critique prévue à l'article L. 5144-1-1 du code de la santé publique et fixant la liste des méthodes de réalisation du test de détermination de la sensibilité des souches bactériennes prévue à l'article R. 5141-117-2*. Journal Officiel de la République Française 2016;0072:3. Available at: https://www.legifrance.gouv.fr/jo_pdf.do?id=JORFTEXT000032291325. [Accessed 9 January 2024].

33. Hayama S. Wildlife Conservation and veterinarians. In: Ikemoto S, Yoshikawa Y, Ito N, editors. Introduction to veterinary science. (Tokyo), Japan: Midorishobou; 2022. p. 98.

34. Ito N. veterinary ethics with wild and exhibit animals. In: Ikemoto S, Yoshikawa Y, Ito N, editors. Animal ethics and animal welfare. Tokyo, Japan: Midorishobou; 2020. p. 126.

35. Available at:The ornithological society of Japan Check list of Japanese birds https://ornithology.jp/katsudo/Publications/Checklist7_e.html. [Accessed 9 January 2024].

36. Japanese Ministry of The Environment. Basic guidelines for implementing projects to protect and manage birds and animals. 2024. Available at: https://

www.env.go.jp/nature/choju/plan/pdf/plan1-1b-R03.pdf. [Accessed 9 January 2024].

37. Forestry and Fisheries. japanese ministry of agriculture japanese veterinarians act. 2024. Available at: https://elaws.e-gov.go.jp/document?lawid=324AC0000000186_20220617_504AC0000000068. [Accessed 9 January 2024].

38. Labour and Welfare. Japanese ministry of health pharmaceutical affairs act 2002. Available at: https://elaws.e-gov.go.jp/document?lawid=335AC0000000145. [Accessed 9 January 2024].

39. Japanese Ministry of The Environment. Act on welfare and management of animals. Available at: 1973 https://elaws.e-gov.go.jp/document?lawid=348AC1000000105_20220617_504AC0000000068. [Accessed 9 January 2024].

40. animal protection index *chapter e: japan.* 2024. Available at: https://api.worldanimalprotection.org/country/japan. [Accessed 9 January 2024].

41. Forestry and Fisheries. Japanese Ministry of Agriculture *Rabies Prevention Act.* 1950. Available at: https://elaws.e-gov.go.jp/document?lawid=325AC1000000247_20160401_426AC000000006. [Accessed 9 January 2024].

42. Labour and Welfare. Japanese ministry of health *act on the prevention of infectious diseases and medical care for patients with infectious Diseases.* 1998. Available at: https://www.japaneselawtranslation.go.jp/ja/laws/view/2830/en. [Accessed 9 January 2024].

43. Japanese ministry of the environment *act on the prevention of Adverse Eçological Impacts Caused by Designated Invasive Alien Species.* 2004. Available at: https://www.env.go.jp/nature/intro/1law/files/20230601_houritsuzenbun.pdf. [Accessed 9 January 2024].

44. Japanese ministry of the environment website *list of regulated living organisms under the invasive alien species Act in Japan.* 2020. Available at: https://www.env.go.jp/nature/intro/2outline/list.html. [Accessed 9 January 2024].

Exotic Animal Practice in Australasia

Hamish R. Baron, BVSc (Hons), MVS (Avian Medicine), PhD, FANZCVS (Avian Medicine and Surgery)*,
James Haberfield, BSc, BVMS, MANZCVS (Unusual Pets, Avian Medicine and Surgery)

KEYWORDS

• Australia • New Zealand • Exotic pet • Avian • Veterinarian • Veterinary profession

KEY POINTS

- The unique avian, reptilian and mammalian biodiversity of Australasia has shaped growth of exotic animal practice in Australasia.
- Many vets and support staff have developed skills in wildlife and conservation medicine which have been translated into pet and companion animal medicine.
- The Australian exotic pet veterinary profession has more dedicated exotic animal veterinary services when compared with the other regions in Australasia.
- Significant growth has occurred in Australasia in both the standards of care and the number of veterinary professionals employed in exotic animal practice, lead by dedicated specialist hospitals and larger exotic pet groups in Australia.
- Veterinarians in general practice, primarily focused on dogs and cats are increasingly recognizing the challenges associated with exotic animal care. Consequently, they are frequently referring such cases to institutions that possess the necessary expertise and resources to ensure optimal care.

INTRODUCTION TO EXOTIC ANIMAL PRACTICE IN AUSTRALASIA

Australasia, comprising Australia, New Zealand, and neighboring Pacific Islands, is a region of unparalleled ecological diversity and unique avian, reptilian, and mammalian species. Australasia is made up of island nations, and the number of endemic species filling specific ecological niches is unparalleled.[1] The islands' geographic isolation, the myriad of endemic species that have found their way into pet homes and breeding collections, combined with strict government legislation makes the Australasian exotic pet veterinary scene truly unique. From its infancy in the early 1960s, to a rapidly growing, dedicated specialist niche, the exotic pet veterinary profession in Australasia

The Unusual Pet Vets, 210 Karingal Drive, VIC 3199, Australia
* Corresponding author.
E-mail address: hamish@unusualpetvets.com.au

Vet Clin Exot Anim 27 (2024) 489–501
https://doi.org/10.1016/j.cvex.2024.03.004
1094-9194/24/© 2024 Elsevier Inc. All rights reserved.
vetexotic.theclinics.com

has morphed into a tight-knit group of passionate veterinarians and support staff practicing medicine and surgery at a high level.

WHAT MAKES AUSTRALASIA UNIQUE?

Australasia's avian, reptilian, and mammalian biodiversity is a testament to the region's unique evolutionary history. From the vibrant plumage of lorikeets and rosellas in Australia to the iconic flightless kakapo and kiwi in New Zealand, this region boasts an array of endemic bird species. These birds have evolved in isolation, adapting to specialized niches and ecosystems. The diversity of Australasian avifauna underscores the delicate ecological balance that has been forged over millions of years. Australasia is home to an array of reptiles that have evolved in isolation, resulting in a fascinating mosaic of adaptations and ecological roles. The frilled-neck lizard of Australia, known for its striking defensive display, and the tuatara of New Zealand, a living fossil representing an ancient lineage, exemplify the remarkable diversity of reptiles in this region. These creatures have not only survived the test of time but have also shaped the ecosystems they inhabit.

New Zealand, owing to its isolation and the lack of mammalian inhabitants when it broke away from Gondwana 80 million years ago, has become a treasure trove of evolutionary novelties.[2] The kiwi, with its vestigial wings and nocturnal habits, alongside a myriad of both extinct and extant flightless native birds that have filled ecological niches that are traditionally filled by mammals throughout the rest of the world.[2] These species have undergone extraordinary adaptations in the absence of mammalian predators, leading to unique ecological roles and behaviors. New Zealand's conservation efforts are intrinsically tied to safeguarding these living relics of evolution, and it is these conservation efforts that have largely been the driving force behind the training and establishment of avian, wildlife, and exotic pet veterinarians in New Zealand.

Australasia's approach to exotic pet ownership is characterized by a dedication to preserving native wildlife and ecosystems. Unlike many other regions, Australia and New Zealand have stringent regulations in place to prevent the introduction of potentially invasive species or diseases. Species that are common throughout the rest of the world, including some birds, rabbits, and ferrets, are subject to restrictions that vary by state or region, while other common exotic pets such as exotic reptiles, chinchillas, hedgehogs, and birds of prey are illegal to own as pets in Australia.[3] Intracountry and intrastate variations further exemplify the nuanced approach taken to address regional ecological concerns. One of the major differences between the Australian and New Zealand management of native species is that Australia forbids the private keeping of any nonnative reptile species, and restricts the ownership of these, as well as many native bird species, to those holding a license.[4] Juxtaposed, is the New Zealand approach, where all native reptiles and birds are illegal to keep as pets, while exotic species are readily available, without permits or licensing requirements.[5] This region-specific legislation provides another layer of complexity in this unique and challenging environment for avian and exotic pet veterinarians.

Australasia's geographic isolation, in conjunction with strict import, export, and licensing laws, has implications for the exotic pet market. The cost to purchase exotic pets in the region often deviates significantly from global averages. In New Zealand, large parrots, and reptiles command high prices due to their scarcity, while in Australia, native parrots that are valued elsewhere are comparatively less expensive. This pricing dynamic reflects the supply and demand, shaping the accessibility of certain species to enthusiasts and collectors. This legislation and border security has also been instrumental in preventing the introduction of exotic diseases such as highly pathogenic avian influenza, West Nile virus, psittacid herpesvirus, and the widespread introduction of avian bornavirus.[6] However, the region is not impervious to risks from smuggling and wildlife migration. Vigilance and stringent biosecurity measures are in place to safeguard the native wildlife and pets from potential threats posed by the inadvertent introduction of foreign species and pathogens.

In Australia, the introduction of wild-caught specimens has led to the rapid establishment of unique morphs in captive populations, particularly in reptiles and birds. This phenomenon has enriched the morphologic diversity of available pets but also raises concerns about the effects of very small founder populations and potential health issues. Unlike some other regions where large businesses control the breeding and sale of exotic pet species, Australasia lacks a structured, commercial breeding industry. This results in a less centralized approach to breeding, with many smaller enthusiasts supplying animals for the exotic pet trade. Consequently, there is less awareness of certain health and disease issues and few controls when it comes to breeding closely related morphologic mutations.

One of the major challenges faced by the exotic pet veterinary profession in Australasia is the lack of dedicated training institutes. While institutions such as Massey University, The University of Sydney, and the University of Queensland offer programs with exposure to exotic pet and wildlife veterinary services through their teaching hospitals, there remain few avenues for veterinary students or veterinarians with ambition to specialize in exotic pet care. The refinement of the veterinary courses at most of the universities in Australasia has led to a reduction in the teaching hours allocated to avian and exotic pets, with many of the courses now focusing solely on "day-one competencies" for small animal and livestock veterinary positions. This has led to a decline in the preparedness and clinical skills of enthusiastic avian and exotic pet-focused graduating veterinarians. It has put the onus on exotic pet employers to provide on-the-job training and introduce these new veterinarians to the skills and knowledge required to treat the diverse range of species seen in exotic pet practice. This significant knowledge gap underscores the need for further investment in education and training for professionals in this field.

The small, close-knit exotic pet veterinary community in Australasia plays a crucial role in the care and welfare of exotic pets. The distance between Australasia and the well-acknowledged leaders in exotic pet veterinary care, Europe and North America, has led to the development of unique training pathways and opportunities for the advancement of skills. The Australian and New Zealand College of Veterinary Scientists (ANZCVS) is a prominent avenue for veterinarians seeking further qualifications in the field. Through the ANZCVS, veterinarians can pursue specialized training and accreditation in Avian Medicine and Surgery, and membership status in Medicine and Surgery of Unusual Pets. This is a common pathway for exotic pet veterinarians to demonstrate a higher level of knowledge. To achieve this qualification, the candidates must have worked for a minimum of 3.5 years following graduation to be eligible to sit the Membership examinations. They are then examined by Members of the Chapter, and if the candidate achieves a pass mark of greater than 70% in each of 3 examinations, they are admitted to the ANZCVS as a Member of their respective chapter. The avian chapter offers Fellowship (Specialist) programs, where the candidate carries out a 2 year residency program, training under 2 other specialists, before being eligible to sit the examinations if they have also met the publication and external training requirements.

Some members of the exotic pet profession in Australia have followed the American or European pathway for specialization, with European or American boarded specialists and a handful of veterinarians with the American Board of Veterinary Practitioners (ABVP) qualification in the Avian or Small Mammal stream practicing in Australia. Those with qualifications from the European College of Zoologic Medicine (ECZM) or American College of Zoologic Medicine have reciprocity and are recognized as specialists in their field, while the ABVP and ANZCVS qualifications are not recognized as specialists outside of their issuing jurisdictions.

Like the ANZCVS, the Association of Avian Veterinarians Australasian Chapter (AAVAC) was started when a group of veterinarians saw a need for cooperation and knowledge-sharing opportunities, with this group paving the way for the collegial nature of the exotic veterinary community. What started as a very small group of passionate larrikins, has helped to shape the ethos of fostering newcomers, fun loving, and having a welcoming spirit that embodies the exotic vet profession in Australasia. These core values were further cemented through the establishment of the Unusual Pets and Avian Vets (UPAV) special interest group of the Australian Veterinary Association, a group that introduced a host of new, keen veterinarians that treated exotic species other than birds. These 2 groups worked alongside and in conjunction with one another, sharing conference venues and dates, resulting in a fun-filled, weeklong dedicated avian and exotic pet conference annually. In recent years, the conferences have occurred in different locations and at different times, but the exotic veterinary community is looking forward to a combined conference again in Canberra in 2024.

The establishment of an exotic pet veterinary community has evolved in Australasia with influence from the rest of the world. Initially, visits from guest speakers, keynote lecturers, and externships carried out by Australasian veterinarians overseas and more recently access to multidiscipline international conferences, virtual conferences, and webinars. Each of these experiences has enriched the community of passionate and dedicated exotic pet veterinarians and helped to shape a truly unique group of professionals.

HISTORICALLY SIGNIFICANT EVENTS

The field of veterinary medicine in Australasia has witnessed a remarkable evolution since the midtwentieth century. As small and mixed animal veterinarians found themselves increasingly presented with unusual and exotic pets for assessment, they embarked on a transformative journey, pushing the boundaries of their knowledge and expertise. We explore the significant events and milestones that have shaped the Australasian exotics veterinary field, decade by decade, shedding light on the pioneers, innovations, and institutions that have played a pivotal role in its development. In the interest of brevity, we have focused on those clinics that exclusively see avian and exotic pet species to try and provide a comprehensive history without discussing nonfoundational small animal practices that have clinicians with an avian and exotic pet caseload.

1960s: the Birth of Avian Medicine

The 1960s marked the birth of avian medicine in Australasia, as veterinarians like Dr Tom Hungerford from Sydney, who published "Diseases of Poultry including Caged Birds and Pigeons" in 1962, laid the foundation for the care of birds.[7] What is now known as the Australasian Veterinary Poultry Association (AVPA) was formed in 1966, further emphasizing the growing interest in avian health.[7] Emerging veterinarians such as Drs Harry Cooper, David Schultz, Garry Cross, Pin Needham, and Ray Butler graduated during this era and pioneered tailored care for exotic pets, primarily focusing on birds.[7] The publication of "Diseases of Cage and Aviary Birds" in 1969, edited by Dr Margaret Petrak, served as a valuable resource for the growing community of avian veterinarians.[7]

1970s: Nurturing Avian and Exotic Expertise

The 1970s saw the nurturing of avian and exotic expertise in Australasia. Dr Michael Raises in Melbourne offered early training courses, passing the baton to Dr David Madill upon his retirement.[7] Graduates like Dr Ross Perry and Dr Rod Reece played pivotal roles in advancing avian medicine.[7] Dr Ross Perry initiated research on psittacine beak and feather disease, a significant contribution to the field. This decade laid the groundwork for further advancements in avian and exotic pet care into the future.

Dr Robert Johnson graduated in 1976 and began his career working for Dr Russell Dickens, and Robert received a large amount of exposure to native mammals during this time, which helped form a foundation for the decades to follow where he would go on to make significant contributions to the field.

1980s: Pioneering Work and Collaborative Growth

The 1980s ushered in a period of pioneering work and collaborative growth within the Australasian exotics veterinary field. As the demand for tailored care for unusual and exotic pets continued to rise, several veterinarians played a pivotal role in shaping the landscape.

Dr Doug Black, who joined forces with Dr David Madill at his Springvale clinic, recounted the challenges and excitement of the era

In the late 1980s and early 1990s, there were very few practicing avian veterinarians in Australia and quite limited reference material. You could say that there was a lot of experimentation and trial and error work happening with all of us. It was a daunting and exciting time, and there were some pioneering vets performing some really innovative work back then. There was also a great willingness of knowledge and experience (both good and bad!) sharing. This was even more so in the ostrich field, where there were probably less than 5 veterinarians worldwide actively involved in ostrich medicine and surgery and virtually no written reference material available. Almost every surgical procedure was done 'for the first time.'
—(Doug Black, personal communication, 2023)

Amid these challenges, the first "Refresher Course on Aviary and Caged Birds" was hosted by the Post Graduate Foundation in Veterinary Science from Sydney University in February 1981, laying the foundation for the future growth of avian medicine in Australia.[8] In 1985, the AVPA hosted a seminar on "Cage and Aviary Bird Medicine," introducing veterinarians to innovations like the use of Isoflurane in avian surgery. One of the members recalled this fondly as

this was the first time we were all "ex- posed" to the wonders of Isoflurane…again a major milestone for avian surgery. I will never forget that sulphur-crested cockatoo recovering after being anaesthetised by Greg Harrison using Isoflurane…we were all gob-smacked!![8]

Dr Garry Cross, who began working at the University of Sydney in 1986, initiated the foundation work on the "Caged Birds" course.[8] Meanwhile, Dr Patricia Macwhirter, who opened the Burwood Bird and Animal Clinic in 1981, published the *Everybird, a Guide to Bird Health* book a few years later.[7]

The 1980s also saw significant contributions from other veterinarians like Dr James Gill, who helped introduce the use of endoscopy for surgical sexing of birds into Australia. James, or Jim as he is often known as, opened Canley Heights Veterinary Hospital in Sydney in 1981, a clinic that is still seeing a lot of exotic animal patients today. Drs Colin Walker, Rob Marshall, and Tony Gestier began treating a large volume of pet birds and ventured into producing aviculture products, including supplements and medications.[7] Notably, Dr Gestier established Vetafarm, now Australia's largest avian pet food manufacturers.

Dr Lucio Filippich, Dr Ross Perry, and Dr Megan Parker made substantial early contributions to the understanding of *Macrorhabdus ornithogaster*. In 1989, Dr Ross Perry became Australia's first registered specialist in Cage and Aviary Birds through what is now known as the ANZCVS. Moreover, the 1980s witnessed the start of expansion into the treatment of more unusual species within the field. Dr Annabelle Olsson began treating crocodiles in Cairns, developing techniques that are still used today. Dr Brendan Carmel embarked on a consulting role for the Ballarat Wildlife Park, paving the way into the realm of zoo and wildlife medicine, with mentorship from Dr Helen McCracken at the Melbourne Zoo. Dr Ray Butler ran a private veterinary clinic in Perth, offering treatment of client-owned nonnative birds and circus animals, including elephants, big cats, bears, and primates, drawing from his experience as the resident veterinarian at the Royal Melbourne Zoo for a decade. Dr David Pass isolated and characterized psittacine beak and feather disease virus through his research at Murdoch University, and he also contributed to the development of the avian medicine lecture course at the university.

Dr Bob Doneley, who had opened his own practice in West Toowoomba in 1988, began building a substantial avian caseload. He fondly recalled these early years in exotics medicine as "*a lot of fun with a small group of like-minded people*" illustrating the camaraderie that defined the community. (Bob Doneley, personal communication, 2023)

These remarkable developments in the 1980s set the stage for further growth and innovation in the field, with veterinarians pushing boundaries and sharing knowledge to meet the evolving needs of unusual and exotic pet owners.

1990s: Collaborations Flourish

In the 1990s, the field of Australasian exotics veterinary care continued to flourish, marked by increased collaboration and specialization. This decade saw the establishment of key organizations and the emergence of dedicated specialists.

The AAVAC, ANZCVS, and the Australian Avian Veterinary Medical Association—a special interest group of the Australian Veterinary Association (AVA)—came together to organize combined annual conferences.[7] These events featured a line-up of international speakers, fostering knowledge exchange and networking opportunities among professionals in the field. The inaugural AAVAC conference in 1992 set a precedent for these collaborative gatherings.

In this decade, Dr Peter Wilson established an exotics veterinary clinic in Currumbin, expanding the resources available in the region for avian and exotic pet care. Meanwhile, Dr Patricia Macwhirter became the second registered specialist in Caged and Aviary Bird Medicine.

Dr Mike Cannon opened the Cannon & Ball Veterinary Surgeons clinic in Wollongong in 1991 and started consulting for several wildlife parks in and around New South Wales. He continued to grow this service and became a Senior Associate teaching the medicine and surgery of birds, reptiles, and small mammals at the University of Sydney in 2005.

Dr Sandy Hume achieved his membership in Avian Health with the ANZCVS in 1993 under the helpful guidance of Dr James Gill. Sandy opened the Canberra Bird Clinic in 1995, bringing some much-needed expertise to the territory. In Far North Queensland, Dr Annabelle Olsson opened Boongarry Veterinary Services in 1993, providing vital veterinary care to both wildlife and unusual pets. Clients from distant locations sought her expertise, reflecting the growing demand for dedicated exotics care. Similarly, in Western Australia, Dr Tim Oldfield was steadily growing his avian and exotic pet caseload. His journey in Australia followed his experience running a 100% avian primary admissions clinic in Durban, South Africa.

Dr Mark Simpson opened the Sugarloaf Animal Hospital in Newcastle in 1994, with a strong focus on unusual, exotic, native, and wildlife patients. Reflecting on the sense of community among veterinarians in the field, he shared

There is a certain sense of it always having been 'my tribe' or my people - a group of veterinarians who share an interest in the same species as me, but for some reason this overflows so that there is significant overlap in many other areas of our outlook on life. Not that we are immune from disagreements or petty jealousy (like any family) but just that in the Venn diagram of life philosophy and outlook, I seem to overlap with these people so much more than any other group in my life.
—(Mark Simpson, personal communication, 2023)

During this time, Dr Danny Brown made significant contributions by producing several husbandry books, offering valuable insights to clinicians and pet owners alike.

The 1990s laid a strong foundation for the continued growth of the exotics veterinary field in Australasia, as professionals came together to share knowledge and enhance care for unusual and exotic pets.

2000s: Exotic Only Veterinary Services and Further Specialization

The 2000s saw the continued emergence of exotic only veterinary services in Australasia. Dr Alex Rosenwax established the Bird and Exotics Veterinarian in Sydney in 2001, one of the first standalone exotics veterinary hospitals in the region. Dr Narelle Price opened the Melbourne Rabbit Clinic in 2006, exclusively dedicated to rabbits and guinea pigs. Dr James Harris, stranded in Tasmania during the 2001 Twin Towers tragedy, decided to stay permanently, establishing a veterinary clinic near Hobart offering avian and exotic veterinary services.[7] In 2003, Dr Phil Sacks became a part owner of the Burwood Bird and Animal Hospital, now known as Bird Vet Melbourne.

Drs Bob Doneley, Deborah Monks, and Shane Raidal attained avian specialist status through the ANZCVS. Dr Monks further achieved recognition through the ECZM after completing her residency under Dr Neil Forbes. Her overseas avian residency broadened her knowledge and exposure, setting the stage for a massive contribution to the profession in Australia over the ensuing decades, having taken on various professional leadership and examination positions since becoming a specialist. In 2006, Dr Monks established the Brisbane Bird and Exotics Veterinary Service, setting the bar for patient care and private exotics veterinary clinical practices in Queensland. Dr Bob Doneley utilized his specialist skills in educating the next generation of veterinarians, taking up a role at The University of Queensland in 2010, where he headed the Avian and Exotic Pet Service, before stepping into a professorial role dedicated to teaching and research. Similarly, Dr Shane Raidal took a role at Charles Sturt University where he has pursued higher education to become a certified Veterinary Pathologist through the ECZM. Dr Raidal has been transformative for the Australasian avian veterinary profession through his contribution to teaching and research, having authored 174 peer-reviewed journal articles and greater than 50 conference proceedings. Many of these publications are formative and have contributed to the understanding of psittacine beak and feather disease on a global scale.

Dr Brendan Carmel continued to build his unusual pet caseload at the Warranwood Veterinary Center in Melbourne. He cofounded the Unusual and Exotic Pets (UEP) Special Interest Group (SIG) of the AVA with Dr Mark Simpson in 2003, providing a more mainstream avenue for general practitioners and exotic pet veterinarians to share knowledge regarding exotic veterinary care. The UEP SIG has evolved into the UPAV SIG, which runs an annual conference that is very well attended by many leading exotic veterinarians in Australia. Dr Sandy Hume had this to say about the importance of UPAV: "*In addition to the AAVAC, the arrival of UPAV was an extremely important development that really led to the maturity of the avian and exotic pet specialty in Australia.*" (Sandy Hume, personal Communication, 2023)

After spending the last few decades building the Springwood Veterinary Clinic in the Blue Mountains of New South Wales and achieving a Certificate in Zoologic Practice with the Royal College of Veterinary Surgeons, Dr Robert Johnson established the South Penrith Veterinary Clinic, which saw a large exotics case load. He also spent time working at Taronga Zoo in Sydney. He summarized the changes he has seen over the course of his career as

> When I graduated there was very little known about the veterinary treatment of exotic species in Australia. Veterinarians prepared to treat these animals were few and far between and the literature was definitely wanting. Today I am impressed by the enthusiasm, knowledge and diligence of emerging and current practitioners. The facilities and equipment available are extraordinary. As pet choices change the veterinary profession must adapt accordingly. In 1976, the year I graduated, the average Australian pet-owning family had a dog, a cat and a bird (usually a canary, budgie, cockatiel, galah or cockatoo). Now our clients expect us to have a good background knowledge in the care of many more species - reptiles, fish, rabbits, Backyard chickens etc.
> —(Robert Johnson, personal communication, 2023)

Dr Shane Simpson has been credited with the advancement of reptile medicine and surgery in Australia, building a substantial reptile caseload at Karingal Vet Hospital in Melbourne. He commented that he observed a significant increase in the number of unusual pets seen in private practice, indicative of a growing demand for expert care. In 2005, Dr David Vella opened an exotics-only service in Sydney within a specialist veterinary hospital, achieving diplomat status with the ABVP in Exotic Companion Mammal Practice. In the same year, Dr Adrian Gallagher opened Brisbane Bird Vet, offering avian-only services, the first of its kind in Queensland.

Dr David Phalen joined the University of Sydney, teaching Exotic and Avian Medicine and revolutionizing the Universities curriculum to prepare graduates for avian and exotic pet practice following graduation.[7] Dr Phalen was instrumental in the establishment of the Avian Reptile and Exotic Pet Hospital and Wildlife Health and Conservation Center, a purpose-built facility in Camden, NSW. This was a state-of-the-art teaching hospital that provided great learning opportunities to Sydney university veterinary students. Working alongside Dr Phalen was Dr Anne Fowler in 2007. When he emigrated to Australia, Dr Phalen also brought his extensive laboratory and diagnostic pathology background with him from the United States. These skills helped to establish many previously unavailable molecular diagnostic tests, which transformed clinical exotic pet practice by facilitating further diagnostic testing and confirmed molecular diagnosis of many viral diseases.

Dr Brett Gartrell emigrated to New Zealand following his work with Adrian Gallagher in Australia during the mid-1990s and was transformative for the avian and exotic pet profession in New Zealand. In 2002, he founded the New Zealand Wildlife Health Center, now known as Wildbase, which is located at Massey University in Palmerston North. The center plays a vital role in providing care to New Zealand's wildlife, but perhaps equally important, providing training opportunities to aspiring wildlife, avian and exotic pet veterinarians. The Wildbase postgraduate residency program has successfully trained numerous residents to achieve membership qualifications with the ANZCVS. Dr Gartrell also shares his expertise by teaching the undergraduate course in avian and reptile medicine and surgery and the postgraduate Master of Veterinary Medicine.

Further north, in Auckland, Dr Kevin Turner purchased the Lynfield Vet Clinic from Berend Westera in 2007 (who subsequently moved to work for Pet Doctors Mount Albert) and opened New Zealand's first privately owned exotics primary accession and referral practice. Reflecting on the journey of exotic pet care in the country, Kevin provided the following summary:

From my observations, the development of the field in New Zealand started around zoo and conservation efforts. Where private clinicians were involved, they took the skills gained back to their practices and applied this to their pet caseload. As the demand for skilled care grew amongst pet owners, the ability to develop referral services developed. Most clinicians were only too happy to send these patients elsewhere.

—*(Kevin Turner, personal communication, 2023)*

Dr Espen Odberg arrived from Norway in 2012 under a special veterinary license to work at Lynfield Vet alongside Dr Turner, treating exotic pet species and together they set about training a group of interns and creating a central hub for exotic pet care in Auckland. However, the Lynfield Veterinary Clinic was sold to Pet Doctors in 2014, and the clinic was merged with Pet Doctors Mt Albert and the flagship clinic Pet Doctors St Lukes & Exotics Centre was formed. Both foundation veterinarians, Dr Westera and Dr Odberg moved on from the clinic shortly afterward, Dr Westera has taken up a role at CareVets Glen Eden where he still sees exotic pets in a part-time capacity, while Dr Odberg has moved back to Norway. Dr Allen Yang has taken over the lead veterinarian role and heads a team of 3 vets who are dedicated to only seeing exotic pet species, out of a larger, multispecies hospital. Meanwhile, Dr Kevin Turner has continued to practice exotic pet medicine in Whangarei out of Mill Road Veterinary Hospital.

The Pacific Islands Veterinary Services was established, providing care for Sea Turtles and other exotic animals in the North Pacific Islands.

2010s: the Continued Growth of Standalone Exotics Clinics

The 2010s marked the rise of the Unusual Pet Vets, founded by Dr James Haberfield in 2012. This group has since grown to become the largest network of exotic animal veterinary clinics in the world.

In early 2013, Dr Gerry Skinner founded the Rabbit Doctors in Melbourne, offering tailored veterinary care to rabbits and guinea pigs. In the same year, Dr Shangzhe Xie established the Avian and Exotic Pet Referral Service at the Adelaide Veterinary Specialist and Referral Center. Dr Jaclyn Gatt and Dr Glynn Lam founded the Bird and Exotic Animal Clinic in Melbourne in 2016, with Dr Anne Fowler opening the Adelaide Bird & Exotics Vet Centre the same year. In 2019, Dr Matthew Gosbell and Dr Patricia Macwhirter purchased the Melbourne Bird Veterinary Clinic from Dr Colin Walker.

In 2016 and 2019, respectively, Drs Melinda Cowan and Hamish Baron became avian specialists through the ANZCVS. Dr Cowan founded an exotics service within a Sydney-based specialist hospital, while Dr Baron became a coowner of the Unusual Pet Vets.

Meanwhile in New Zealand, Dr Lisa Argilla completed her residency at Massey University in New Zealand, achieving membership-level qualifications in Avian Health through the ANZCVS in 2010. She started an independent consultancy service, which eventually evolved into the Dunedin Wildlife Hospital, further expanding the spectrum of care for wildlife and exotic species in New Zealand's South Island.

Dr Tim Hyndman, a distinguished researcher at Murdoch University, made significant contributions to our understanding of reptile pathogens throughout the 2010s, with a particular focus on viruses. His groundbreaking research on Sunshine virus has not only advanced our current knowledge but also laid the foundation for future research in this critical field. Dr Hyndman's unwavering commitment to unraveling the complexities of reptile viruses is truly remarkable and deserves utmost recognition.

The first Association of Reptile and Amphibian Veterinarians conference in the Southern Hemisphere took place in Cairns in April 2014. This milestone event significantly enhanced the awareness and engagement of Australian veterinarians within the broader global community of reptile veterinary professionals.

2020 to 2023: Advancing Avian Specialization

In 2021 and 2023, Drs Alex Mastakov and Michelle Sutherland became avian specialists through the ANZCVS, bringing the total number of Avian Fellows in Australasia to 8, the most registered specialists ever. At the time of writing, there are several residents currently undergoing specialist training but are yet to credential for examinations.

In 2022, Dr Robert Johnson became a Member of the Order of Australia (AM) in recognition of the significant service to veterinary science and to professional societies. This is an incredible honor that is only awarded to a very select number of people.

Several new exotics only services have opened in Australia during the early 2020s including The Exotics Vet in Brisbane headed up by Dr Vanessa Harkess, Exotics Services at the Veterinary Specialists of Sydney headed up by Dr Dean Felker, and the Avian & Exotics Service in The Pet Specialists, Sydney, headed up by Dr Izidora Sladakovic.

Meanwhile in New Zealand, Dr Martin Earles opened the Tauranga Exotic Vet in 2021 that, together with Dr Allen Yang and his team at Pet Doctors St Lukes & Exotics Centre in Auckland, is helping to make expert exotic pet care more accessible.

LIKELY FUTURE TRAJECTORY
Australia

Australia's exotic pet landscape is undergoing a transformative shift, marked by the aging of the single vet trailblazers who helped establish exotic animal care in Australia, the rise of prominent market players and the establishment of specialized services within multidisciplinary hospitals. This evolution is further fueled by the changing dynamics of pet ownership, increasing urbanization, and a growing demand for high-quality care for exotic animals. Some of the key likely future trajectory ideas are explored in the following sections.

Retirement of Single Vet, Small Exotic Pet Practice Owners

One of the primary driving forces shaping the future of exotic animal veterinary services in Australia is the retirement of single vet, small exotic pet practice owners.

Many of these pioneers who initially established practices to cater to the unique needs of exotic pets are nearing retirement age. As they contemplate exiting the profession, the challenge lies not only in passing on the knowledge and experience gained over the years but also in maintaining the personalized care that has become a hallmark of these practices. The retirement of these practitioners opens the door for new entrants to take on the responsibility of caring for Australia's exotic pet population and provides potential pathways for practice ownership to employees of these practices.

Rise of Larger Market Players

In response to the changing landscape, larger market players like The Unusual Pet Vets have emerged as prominent contributors to the future trajectory of exotic animal veterinary services in Australia. These clinics, with multiple locations across the country, are strategically positioned to provide continuity of care for clients as well as opportunities for continued employment when staff members relocate. The scale of operations and the ability to invest in advanced facilities, processes, and technologies position them as leaders in exotic animal care and employment standards. The larger infrastructure allows for collaboration, knowledge sharing, and the development of specialized skills. Having a larger group in the exotic pet veterinary space has brought about a shift in employee expectations, with a transition toward exotic pet veterinarians reaching parity or better with their traditional small animal veterinary counterparts when it comes to employment conditions and career opportunities. As the demand for exotic pet care increases, these clinics are well equipped to expand their services, hire specialized staff, and contribute to the professional development of veterinarians with an interest in exotic species.

Specialized Services within Larger Hospitals

Another noteworthy trend in the future trajectory of exotic animal veterinary services in Australia is the integration of specialized services within multidisciplinary hospitals. Recognizing the unique needs of exotic pets, facilities like the Small Animal Specialist Hospital in Sydney, the Northside Veterinary Specialists in Sydney, the Veterinary Specialists of Sydney, and the University of Queensland are opening complementary exotic services within their existing infrastructure. This integration not only provides access to state-of-the-art facilities and equipment but also facilitates collaboration between general practitioners, emergency critical care, and multidisciplinary specialists. Exotic pets that may require a combination of expertise can now receive comprehensive care within a single institution. The collaboration between specialized services and other services within multidisciplinary hospitals sets a new standard for exotic animal care and reflects the evolving expectations of clients. These collaborations will undoubtedly lead to an improvement in patient care and the development of improved surgical and medical outcomes that continue to advance our understanding of what is possible in exotic pet medicine.

Increasing Exotic Pet Ownership in Australia

The landscape of pet ownership in Australia is evolving, driven by factors such as urbanization and changing family dynamics. As block sizes get smaller and families seek pets that fit into compact living spaces, exotic animals are gaining popularity as "low maintenance pets." Species like reptiles, birds, and small mammals are finding their way into households, contributing to a diverse range of pets beyond traditional cats and dogs.

Referral Practices and Second Opinions

The historical attitude of approaching exotic pet care with a generalist mindset is becoming outdated. Clients now expect higher standards of care for their exotic pets and are willing to invest in high-level veterinary services. Veterinarians caring for exotic pets are now expected to meet elevated standards, reflecting a growing acknowledgment of the intricate and varied care demanded by different species. Consequently, there is a notable surge in both veterinarians and veterinary nurses seeking advanced training and certifications in exotic animal medicine. The accessibility and comprehensiveness of continuing education courses have also improved, making them more available to professionals looking to enhance their expertise in this field.

Veterinarians in general practice, primarily focused on dogs and cats, are increasingly recognizing the challenges associated with exotic animal care. Consequently, they are frequently referring such cases to institutions that possess the necessary expertise and resources to ensure optimal care. Furthermore, clients are more likely to seek a second opinion if their exotic pet is facing a challenging medical condition and they are not satisfied with the care they have received. This trend highlights a shift in client awareness and a growing demand for comprehensive and expert care, even in cases where the primary diagnosis has been established. This shift is also increasingly apparent in the changing perspectives of veterinary surgeon boards, as they emphasize the growing significance of possessing sufficient knowledge and skills in exotic animal medicine for clinicians opting to treat these species.

New Zealand

Anticipated to mirror the trends observed in Australia, New Zealand is poised to undergo a comparable evolution in its veterinary services for exotic animals, albeit at a more gradual pace. The prevalence of exotic pet ownership in New Zealand does not match that of Australia, and the regulatory framework imposes stricter limitations on the types of animal's clients are permitted to keep.

Pacific Islands

The ongoing scarcity of veterinary services in the Pacific Islands is expected to continue in the foreseeable future. With a limited number of exotic pets in the region, it is unlikely that there will be a significant demand for numerous veterinary clinicians. The distinct features of the Pacific Islands imply that the veterinary scene will probably maintain a more modest presence, and tailored care for exotic pets is likely to remain relatively uncommon.

SUMMARY

The diverse and unparalleled ecological landscape of Australasia has forged a unique environment for exotic animal practice, characterized by its rich biodiversity and stringent legislation. From its origins in the 1960s to its current status as a dedicated specialist niche, the exotic pet veterinary profession in Australasia has undergone a remarkable evolution.

The profession faces hurdles in education and training, with limited dedicated institutes offering comprehensive programs, leading to a knowledge gap that employers must bridge. However, the close-knit community of passionate veterinarians has forged unique training pathways and opportunities, establishing a vibrant and highly skilled group of professionals.

The historical timeline showcases pivotal events and influential figures who laid the foundation for the field's growth, decade by decade, from the birth of avian medicine to the establishment of dedicated veterinary clinics. The collaborative efforts and pioneering work of veterinarians have continually propelled the field forward, shaping it into what it is today.

Looking ahead, the landscape of exotic animal veterinary services in Australasia is poised for transformation. The retirement of trailblazers heralds a shift in ownership, while larger market players and specialized services within multidisciplinary hospitals are poised to lead the way. Increasing exotic pet ownership and evolving client expectations emphasize the need for specialized care and elevated standards in the field.

As the demand for specialized care grows, the profession faces the challenge of meeting these evolving expectations while ensuring continued access to advanced training and resources. The future trajectory sees a convergence of specialized services, increased collaboration, and a recognition of the intricate care demands of exotic pets, ultimately driving the field toward higher standards. The hope is that through all of these changes, the profession can maintain its sense of collegiality, companionship, and sense of enjoyment that have been hallmarks of the exotic pet veterinary community since its inception.

DISCLOSURE

The authors are both part owners and directors of The Unusual Pet Vets clinics in Australia as well as current Presidents of the Avian Chapter (Dr H.R. Baron), and the Unusual Pets Chapter (Dr J. Haberfield) of the ANZCVS.

REFERENCES

1. Chapman AD. Numbers of living species in Australia and the world. Australian Biological Resources Study. Australia: Canberra; 2009.
2. Worthy TH, De Pietri VL, Scofield RP. Recent advances in avian palaeobiology in New Zealand with implications for understanding New Zealand's geological, climatic and evolutionary histories. N Z J Zool 2017;44:177–211.
3. Victoria A. Unique or exotic pets. 2023. Available at: https://www.agriculture.gov.au/biosecurity-trade/travelling/bringing-mailing-goods/unique-exotic-pets. [Accessed 2 January 2024].
4. Victoria A. Private wildlife licence. 2023. Available at: https://www.vic.gov.au/private-wildlife-licences. [Accessed 2 January 2024].
5. Service NZC. Bringing pets and animals into New Zealand. 2023. Available at: https://www.customs.govt.nz/personal/move-to-nz-permanently/import-pets-and-animals/. [Accessed 2 January 2024].
6. Australian Department of Agriculture WatE. Import risk review for psittacine birds from all countries – draft review. Canberra: Australian Department of Agriculture, Water and the Environment; 2000.
7. Macwhirter P. Development of avian medicine in Australia. Australian Veterinary History Record 2013;64:20–8.
8. Cross GM. The formation of an association of avian veterinarians in Australia. Part A. AAVAC Newsletter May 2015. Sydney, Australia: Association of Avian Veterinarians Australasian Committee; 2015. p. 1–5.

Exotic Animal Practice in East Asia

A Retrospective Study of Species Distribution and Their Common Diseases at 2 Exotics-only Veterinary Clinics in the East Asia Region

Katerina C.L. Leung, BSc(Vet) (Hons I), BVSc (Hons I)[a],*,
Jeremy Z.F. Kan, BVSc (Hons I)[a,1], Wen-Lin Wang, DVM, MS[b,2]

KEYWORDS

- Bird • Psittacine • Small mammals • Rabbit • Reptile • Veterinary medicine
- Hong Kong • Taiwan

KEY POINTS

- The similarities and differences in the variety and prevalence of different species and their common disorders of patients presented to 2 avian-and-exotics-only clinics in the East Asia region were identified and discussed in this study.
- Exotic companion mammals were the most common class of exotic patients in Hong Kong, while birds appeared to be the most common unconventional patients in Taiwan.
- The most common type of birds presented were small-to-medium-sized parrots, while rabbits and testudines were the most common exotic companion mammals and reptiles presented to avian-and-exotics-only practices in the East Asia region respectively.
- Owners preferences towards veterinary treatment and welfare-related issues of unconventional pets were also identified in the study, further studies are required to address these knowledge gaps.

INTRODUCTION

Throughout the years, a number of retrospective clinical studies have been performed by veterinarians from different exotic animal practices around the world.[1–5] Some of these studies projected a general overview of species prevalence among all patients presented,[1,2] while others described the range of pathologies diagnosed in certain

[a] Concordia Pet Care; [b] Brave Vet Exotic Animal Veterinary Hospital
[1] Present address. LG & P1, No. 5-7 Blue Pool Road, Happy Valley, Hong Kong
[2] Present address. No 227, Minquan W Rd Datong Dist, Taipei City, 103041, Taiwan.
* Corresponding author.
E-mail address: cleu8644@alumni.sydney.edu.au

Vet Clin Exot Anim 27 (2024) 503–519
https://doi.org/10.1016/j.cvex.2024.03.005
1094-9194/24/© 2024 Elsevier Inc. All rights reserved.
vetexotic.theclinics.com

class or species, such as birds,[3] guinea pigs,[4] and bearded dragons.[5] Collectively, these articles highlighted the common diseases affecting some of the popular exotic animal species in the American and European countries.

Similar retrospective studies have been published in the East Asia region, yet mostly only targeted on either a single type of disease[6] or one particular species.[7] A combination of both was investigated in some more recent studies in Taiwan, for example, the prevalence of polyomavirus and circovirus infection in parrots[8] and that of dermatophytosis in rabbits.[9] Shiga and colleagues once performed a study in Japan, investigating the prevalence of neoplastic diseases in exotic companion mammals (ECM), yet only 4 selected species were covered in the study.[10]

With surveys performed in Hong Kong and Taiwan estimating more than 25.0% of pets owned by members of public belonging being birds and exotic species,[11,12] along with the increase toward demand of exotics-only practices in Japan,[13] it is deduced that there is a significant demand for veterinary services exclusively for avian and exotic companion animals. However, retrospective clinical studies providing a general overview of species prevalence in exotics-only practices, or that describing the diseases often diagnosed in common avian and exotic species, remained relatively sparse compared to American and European countries.

The aim of this retrospective clinical study was to describe the variety and prevalence of different species and their common disorders of patients presented to 2 avian-and-exotics-only clinics in the East Asia region (Hong Kong and Taiwan) over a 1 year period, in an attempt to obtain an insight toward the current clinical situation of 2 exotics-only referral practices in the area.

MATERIALS AND METHODS
Case Selection and Classification

Retrospective data were retrieved from the medical records of the Exotics Services Department of the Concordia Pet Care (CPC), Happy Valley, Hong Kong and the Section of Large Animal Disease and Economic Animal Disease, National Taiwan University Veterinary Hospital (NTUVH), Taipei City, Taiwan over a 12 month period from December 2022 to November 2023, as these exotic departments were regarded as high-quality referral practices within their respective country that are equipped with advanced veterinary practitioners in the field (CPC was led by a triple-boarded specialist, while National Taiwan University Veterinary Hospital [NTUVH] was headed by a professor) along with latest equipment and supplies.

Only patients involved in new cases were included in this study. Follow-up consultations were considered as part of the same case and were omitted from being counted toward the study, while returning patients being seen for new problems were included as a new case.

One thousand one hundred eighty-three cases met the inclusion criteria and had complete clinical records for assessment.

Patients presented were grouped according to their taxonomic class and order, under avian, reptile, and ECM. Species that did not fall under the broader categories were categorized as "Others." Avian patients were all patients under the taxonomic class Aves, while reptilian patients were of those class Reptilia. According to the list of recognized veterinary specialties made by the American Board of Veterinary Practitioners, ECM included small mammal species that are commonly kept as pets, including rabbits, rodents, ferrets, hedgehogs, and sugar gliders.[14]

Cases were classified according to organ systems affected by the disease(s) diagnosed. Patients that were presented for general health checks or routine procedures were classified as "clinically healthy"; while cases with no definitive diagnoses were classified as "open diagnosis." Due to neoplasms having the potential to affect multiple organ systems (ie, metastasis and paraneoplastic disease), undiagnosed masses were classified as "mass with unknown nature and origin." Cases that were complex, involving multiple systems, were also noted.

Data Collection and Statistical Analysis

Data were extracted from the medical records and subsequently analyzed with Microsoft Excel, Version 16.58 in Hong Kong. All percentages calculated were corrected to 1 decimal place.

RESULTS
Overview

During the 1 year period from December 01, 2022 to November 30, 2023, a total of 1183 cases were presented to the Exotics Services Department of the CPC in Hong Kong and the Section of Large Animal Disease and Economic Animal Disease at the NTUVH in Taipei, Taiwan. The number of diagnoses made differ to that of cases, as multiple pathologies were diagnosed in 161 cases (13.6%; **Table 1**).

Hong Kong

Birds
One hundred twenty-seven birds were presented over the 12 month period, with vast majority (96.7%) of them belonging to the order Psittaciformes. The remaining cases were made up of Passeriformes (1.6%), with occasional Anseriformes (0.8%) and Columbiformes (0.8%).

The most common type of case seen relates to the gastrointestinal tract, such as gastroenteritis and metal toxicity, accounting for one-fifth (20.5%) of the total cases presented. Skin and musculoskeletal disorders followed as the second and third-most commonly encountered cases in this class (**Table 2**).

One-fifth (20.5%) of avian cases did not achieve a diagnosis (**Table 3**). The monk parakeet (*Myiopsitta monachus*) was the most common species (13.8%) of all avian patients presented. This species was mostly diagnosed with gastrointestinal tract diseases (41.2%), dermatologic disorders (23.5%), or cases with open diagnoses (17.6%). Thirteen lovebirds (*Agapornis* sp) made up 10.6% of all bird cases, making them the second-most common bird species presented. Musculoskeletal disorders were diagnosed in 38.5% of the patients, followed by dermatologic disorders and open diagnoses as both of these diagnoses were seen in 23.1% of lovebird cases, respectively.

Exotic Companion Mammals
Overview. ECM accounted for the largest group of exotic animals seen, with 761 cases over the selected 1 year timeframe (**Fig. 1**). Rabbits (*O cuniculus*) were most frequently presented, accounting for 51.5% ECM cases, followed by Chinchillas

Table 1		
Total number of cases presented to Concordia Pet Care and National Taiwan University Veterinary Hospital and number of cases diagnosed with multiple disorders		
	CPC	NTUVH
Total no. of cases	1013	176
No. of cases diagnosed with multiple disorders (%)	133 (13.1%)	28 (15.9%)

Table 2
Top 5 presumptive pathologies diagnosed in different exotic pets presented to Concordia Pet Care

Class	Order/Group	Presumptive Pathology	Example of Diagnoses	Prevalence of Diagnosis (%)
Avian	—	Gastrointestinal disorders	Gastroenteritis, metal toxicity, and avian bornaviral ganglioneuritis	20.5
		Open diagnosis	—	20.5
		Skin disorders	Dermatitis, feather-picking, and open wound	19.7
		Musculoskeletal disorders	Fracture and joint dislocation	18.1
		Respiratory disorders	Pneumonia, rhinitis, and sinusitis	9.4
ECM	Rabbit	Musculoskeletal disorders	Fractures, pododermatitis, and herniation	15.1
		Clinically healthy	—	12.5
		Respiratory disorders	Rhinitis, pneumonia, and thoracic abscess	11.5
		Dental diseases	Dental/facial abscess and malocclusion	11.2
		Open diagnosis	—	11.0
ECM	Guinea pig	Dental diseases	Dental abscess, overgrown teeth, and malocclusion	22.1
		Musculoskeletal disorders	Fracture, open wound, and pododermatitis	16.2
		Urinary tract disorders	Cystitis, urolith, and renal disease	14.7
		Skin disorders	Dermatitis, fur loss, and broken nail	11.8
		Clinically healthy	—	10.3
ECM	Chinchilla	Clinically healthy	—	22.5
		Dental diseases	Dental abscess, teeth overgrowth, and malocclusion	14.7
		Open diagnosis	—	14.7
		Musculoskeletal disorders	Fracture, soft tissue swelling, and open wound	14.0
		Eye disorders	Conjunctivitis, corneal ulcer, and glaucoma	14.0
ECM	Hamster	Skin disorders	Dermatitis, ectoparasites, skin abscess, and skin mass	17.2
		Open diagnosis	—	13.9
		Mass of unknown origin	—	13.1
		Reproductive disorders	Vaginal bleeding, uterine mass, and ovarian cysts	11.5
		Eye disorders	Conjunctivitis, corneal ulcer, and Harderian gland abscess	8.2

Reptiles	Testudines	Open diagnosis	—	22.4
		Skin disorders	Shell rot, open wound, and broken nail	19
		Musculoskeletal disorders	Fracture, deformed shell, and osteoporosis	17.2
		Urinary tract disorders	Renal disease, gout, and renal tumor	12.1
		Gastrointestinal disorders	Foreign body, constipation, and diarrhea	8.6
Reptiles	Squamata	Open diagnosis	—	20.4
		Reproductive disorders	Follicular stasis, dystocia, hemipenis prolapse, and necrosis	14.3
		Gastrointestinal disorders	Endoparasites, foreign body, and cloacal/colon prolapse	14.3
		Skin disorders	Skin abscess and open wound	12.2
		Eye disorders	Conjunctivitis and anisocoria	10.2
		Musculoskeletal disorders	Tail injury or necrosis and spinal fracture	10.2

Table 3
List of avian species presented at Concordia Pet Care between December 01, 2022 and November 30, 2023

Order	Species
Psittaciformes	African gray parrot (*Psittacus erithacus*), Amazon parrot (*Amazona* spp), budgerigar (*M undulatus*), Caique (*Pionites* sp), cockatiel (*N hollandicus*), galah (*Eolophus roseicapilla*), Moluccan cockatoo (*Cacatua moluccensis*), sulphur-crested cockatoo (*Cacatua galerita*), umbrella cockatoo (*C alba*), yellow-crested cockatoo (*C sulphurea*), Conures, Dusky parrot (*Pionus fuscus*), Moluccan eclectus (*Eclectus roratus*), golden parakeet (*Guaruba guarouba*), Jardine parrot (*Poicephalus gulielmi*), lovebirds (*Agapornis* sp), red-and-green macaw (*Ara chloropterus*), red-shouldered macaw (*Diopsittaca nobilis*), golden-collared macaw (*Primolius auricollis*), blue-and-gold macaw (*Ara ararauna*), monk parakeet (*M monachus*), Pacific parrotlet (*Forpus coelestis*), ringneck parakeet (*Psittacula krameria*), and Senegal parrot (*Poicephalus senegalus*)
Anseriformes	Duck
Columbiformes	Dove
Passeriformes	Java sparrow (*Padda oryzivora*) and myna

(*Chinchilla lanigera*, 17.0%), Hamsters (Cricetinae, 15.9%), and Guinea pigs (*Cavia porcellus*, (8.9%); **Table 4**).

Rabbits. A total of 392 rabbits were seen at CPC throughout the selected 1 year period, making it the most common species presented to the clinic as it accounted for 38.7% of all cases and more than half (51.5%) of ECM cases.

Ten types of rabbits were seen at the clinic throughout the year. Dwarf rabbits accounted for nearly one-third (32.0%) of all rabbits presented and 12.4% of all cases, making them the most common group of rabbits and exotic patients seen at the clinic overall. Lop rabbits were the second-most common group of rabbits presented (27.0%), followed by Lion Head Rabbits (24.4%). For 1.5% of rabbits, the exact group or breed was not specified.

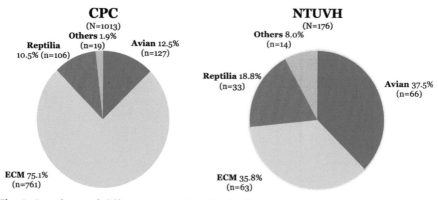

Fig. 1. Prevalence of different categories of animals presented to Concordia Pet Care and National Taiwan University Veterinary Hospital between December 01, 2022 and November 30, 2023.

Order	Species
Table 4	
List of exotic companion mammals species presented at Concordia Pet Care between December 01, 2022 and November 30, 2023	
Lagomorpha	Rabbit (*O cuniculus*)
Rodentia	Guinea pigs (*C porcellus*), chinchillas, (*C lanigera*), hamsters (Cricetinae), fancy rat (*R norvegicus domestica*), mouse, squirrel (Sciuridae), fat-tailed gerbil (*Pachyuromys duprasi*), chipmunk, and prairie dog (*Cynomys* spp)
Carnivora	Ferret (*Mustela furo*) and mongoose (Herpestidae)
Eulipotyphla	North African hedgehog (*Atelerix algirus*) and 4 toed hedgehog (*A albiventris*)
Others	Sugar glider (*P breviceps*)

The most common diagnosis made in rabbits were musculoskeletal disorders (15.1%), predominated by fractures, followed by "clinically healthy" (12.5%) and respiratory issues (11.5%); see **Table 2**.

Guinea pigs. Guinea pigs made up 6.7% of all cases and 8.9% of ECM cases. The most common diagnoses seen in these guinea pigs were dental diseases (22.1%), followed by musculoskeletal disorders (16.2%) and diseases of the urinary tract (4.7%; see **Table 2**).

Chinchillas. Chinchillas accounted for 12.7% of all cases admitted to CPC, hence the second-most commonly seen ECM species at the clinic. More than one-fifth of these chinchillas were diagnosed as "clinically healthy." Dental diseases and "open diagnosis" ranked equally as the second-most common diagnoses in the species, with each being observed in 14.7% chinchilla cases, respectively. Musculoskeletal and ocular disorders were both seen as the third-most common diagnoses, each contributed to the clinical pathologies of 14.0% chinchillas (see **Table 2**).

Hamsters. Hamsters amounted to 122 cases seen, which made up 12.0% of all cases throughout the year analyzed. They are also the third mostly encountered group of ECM at the clinic as they contributed to 16.0% of these cases. The majority (70.2%) of hamsters presented was golden hamsters (*Mesocricetus auratus*), followed by dwarf hamsters (24.8%), while the remaining 5.0% were all Roborovski hamsters (*Phodopus roborovskii*).

Dermatologic pathology was most commonly diagnosed in these animals (17.2%), followed by cases with open diagnoses (13.9%) and space-occupying mass with unknown nature or origin (13.1%; see **Table 2**).

Other exotic companion mammals. There were 50 (6.6%) patients that fell into the category of ECM, but they did not belong to the major species listed above. Approximately half (50.8%) of these were hedgehogs (Erinaceinae), 18.0% were sugar gliders (*Petaurus breviceps*), and 11.5% were fancy rats (*Rattus norvegicus domestica*). The full list of other ECM species presented and the range of diagnoses seen in these patients were listed in **Table 3**.

Reptiles

Cases of reptiles amounted to 106 at CPC during the 12 month period studied, which was equivalent to 10.5% of all total cases. The reptilian cases were near-equally shared by patients from 2 orders, with Testudines taking up a slightly greater share of 54.7%, while the remaining 45.3% being taken by animals from the order of Squamata (**Table 5**).

Testudines. With more than one-fifth of all 58 turtles and tortoises presented to the clinic having an open diagnosis, pathologies of the skin became the second-most common in these patients, as it was observed in nearly one-fifth (19.0%) of Testudines. The third and fourth-most diagnosed categories of pathologies belonged to that of the musculoskeletal system (17.2%) and urinary tract (12.1%; see **Table 2**).

Red-eared sliders (*Trachemys scripta elegans*) accounted for 43.1% of all Testudines presented, making them the most common species among all turtles and tortoises, as well as that of the all reptilian patients seen at the clinic. Diseases of the urinary tract and musculoskeletal system were most commonly diagnosed in the species, as each of these pathologies was diagnosed in 20.0% of cases.

Squamata. Similar to that observed in patients belonging to the order of Testudines, approximately one-fifth (20.8%) of scaled reptiles presented were diagnosed as open cases. Reproductive and gastrointestinal pathologies were equally seen as the most commonly diagnosed disorders in these animals, with diseases belonging to these categories diagnosed in 14.6% of cases, followed by musculoskeletal and ocular diseases that were also seen in 10.4% of patients, respectively (see **Table 2**).

More than one-third of patients from this order were bearded dragons (*Pogona* spp), and they made up 16.0% of reptile cases. No diagnoses were achieved in a significant proportion of these animals (41.2%). Gastrointestinal pathologies were diagnosed in nearly a quarter (23.5%) of all bearded dragons presented, while neurologic issues were seen in 11.8%.

Leopard gecko (*Eublepharis macularius*) was the second-most presented group of scaled reptiles at the clinic. The most common diagnoses seen in these patients were reproductive pathologies (38.5%), followed by skin diseases (23.1%) and ocular abnormalities (15.4%).

Other species. Eight (0.8%) out of all cases seen at CPC were patients who did not fall under any of the above 3 major categories. Half (50%) of these were amphibians, while another 3 (37.5%) were primates, all belonging to the genus of slow lories (*Nycticebus* sp). The remaining patient was a kinder goat (*Capra aegagrus hircus*). The list of these "other" patients and their diagnoses are listed in the following table (**Table 6**).

Table 5
List of reptilian species presented at Concordia Pet Care between December 01, 2022 and November 30, 2023

Order	Species
Testudines	Chinese pond turtle (*Mauremys reevesii*), Chinese stripe-necked turtle (*M sinensis*), golden coin turtle (*C trifasciata*), diamond back terrapin (*Malaclemys terrapin*), map turtle (*Graptemys* sp), musk turtle (Kinosternidae), red-eared slider (*T scripta elegans*), yellow-bellied slider (*Trachemys scripta scripta*), yellow pond turtle (*Mauremys mutica*), and yellow-spotted amazon river turtle (*Podocnemis unifilis*)
	Hermann's tortoise (*Testudo hermanni*), leopard tortoise (*S pardalis*), red-footed tortoise (*Chelonoidis carbonarius*), and African spurred tortoise (*C sulcata*)
Squamata	Bearded dragon (*Pogona* spp), blue tegu, red tegu, blue-tongued skink (*Tiliqua* sp), chameleon (Chamaeleonidae), crested gecko (*Correlophus ciliates*), frilled lizard (*Correlophus ciliatus*), gecko, common iguana (*I iguana*), and leopard gecko (*E macularius*)
	Ball python (*Python regius*), corn snake (*P guttatus*), and hognose

Table 6
List of other species presented to Concordia Pet Care between December 01, 2022 and November 30, 2023 and their presumptive pathologies

Class of Patient	Order of Patient	Patient genus/Species	Presumptive Pathologies
Amphibia	Anura	Bushveld rain frog (*Breviceps adspersus*)	Eye disorders
		Horned frog (*Ceratophrys ornata*)	Gastrointestinal disorders Gastrointestinal disorders Open diagnosis
Mammalia	Artiodactyla	*Capra*	Musculoskeletal + neurologic disorders
	Primate	*Nycticebus* sp	Dental diseases Skin disorders Open diagnosis

Taiwan

Birds

Patients from the class Aves represented 66 of all 176 cases (37.5%) seen at NTUVH, making them the most commonly presented class of animals at the hospital during the timeframe analyzed. While more than half (62.1%) of these patients belonged to the order Psittaciformes, the remaining birds were from a range of other orders, namely the Passeriformes (13.6%), Anseriformes (9.0%), Columbiformes (7.6%), Galliformes (6.1%), and Piciformes (1.5%).

The most commonly diagnosed pathologies in birds were musculoskeletal (21.2%), dermatologic (19.7%), and gastrointestinal (16.7%) diseases (**Table 7**).

Lovebirds (*Agapornis* sp) and cockatiels (*Nymphicus hollandicus*) were the most common species of birds presented to NTUVH throughout the year, as they both amount to 10.6% of all avian cases. 28.6% of all lovebirds were diagnosed with issues of the skin, making such the most commonly observed abnormality in the species, while more than half (57.1%) of all cockatiels seen at the hospital was found to be clinically healthy.

Table 7
List of Avian species presented at National Taiwan University Veterinary Hospital between December 01, 2022 and November 30, 2023

Order	Species
Psittaciformes	African gray parrot (*P erithacus*), budgerigar (*M undulatus*), Caique (*Pionites* sp), cockatiel (*N hollandicus*), African gray parrot (*P erithacus*), Amazon parrot (*Amazona* spp), budgerigar (*M undulatus*), caique (*Pionites* sp), cockatiel (*N hollandicus*), blue-eyed cockatoo (*Cacatua ophthalmica*), umbrella cockatoo (*C alba*), Conures, Moluccan eclectus (*E roratus*), golden parakeet (*G guarouba*), lorikeet (*Loriini* sp), lovebirds (*Agapornis* sp), macaw, monk parakeet (*M monachus*), Pacific parrotlet (*F coelestis*), and Bourke's parrot (*Neopsephotus bourkii*)
Passeriformes	Java sparrow (*L oryzivora*), myna, and Oriental magpie (*Pica serica*)
Anseriformes	Duck, goose, and Brown Tsaiya duck (*Anas platyrhynchos*)
Columbiformes	Pigeon and white-bellied green pigeon (*Treron sieboldii*)
Galliformes	Chicken and Japanese Bantam
Piciformes	Black-browed barbet (*Psilopogon oorti*)

The second-most presented species of birds were the budgerigars (*Melopsittacus undulatus*) and the Java sparrow (*Lonchura oryzivora*). No definitive diagnoses were achieved in one-third (33.3%) of all budgerigar cases presented, while dermatologic abnormalities were detected in another one-third (33.3%) of this species. For the Java sparrows, a range of diseases in the reproductive, gastrointestinal, and respiratory tract, along with pathologies of the eye, musculoskeletal system, and mass of unknown origin were diagnosed in this species in an equal proportion.

Exotic companion mammals
Overview. ECM made up 35.8% of all cases that were presented to the NTUVH, making them the second-most common class of patients brought the hospital. Majority of these patients were rabbits (58.7%), while the others were mainly of "other ECM" and guinea pigs (12.7%) (**Table 8**).

Rabbits. Thirty-seven rabbits were seen at the NTUVH, which attributed to more than one-fifth of the total cases and made it the most common species at the clinic. Six breeds of rabbits were recorded, with 29.7% of these being Dutch rabbits, while the others are New Zealand White rabbits, Siamese rabbits, dwarf rabbits, and lop rabbits. For more than half (54.0%) of the rabbit patients, the exact breed was not recorded.

The most disorders diagnosed made in these rabbits were dental diseases (21.6%), neurologic disorders (16.2%), and musculoskeletal issues (13.5%), respectively.

Guinea pigs. Guinea pigs were found to be the third-most commonly presented ECM species, as they accounted 12.7% cases in this class of patients. This species also accounted for 4.5% of all cases seen at the hospital during the timeframe analyzed. Lymphoma was categorized as a lymphoid disorder in this study and was the most commonly diagnosed disease in these animals, while a range of other pathologies were also observed in these patients.

Chinchillas. Two chinchillas were seen throughout the timeframe analyzed. Pathologies of the central nervous system were seen in both chinchillas presented, while 1 of the 2 also suffered from musculoskeletal disorders due to fracture of the spine in the lumbar region.

Hamster. A total of 4 hamsters were presented to the hospital. Half (50%) of these patients were golden hamsters, while the other half (50.0%) were winter white dwarf hamsters (*Phodopus sungorus*). Dermatologic diseases were diagnosed in half (50%) of the hamsters, while the remaining 2 were found to be affected by gastrointestinal pathologies and a space-occupying lesion of unknown origin, respectively.

Table 8
List of exotic companion mammals species presented at National Taiwan University Veterinary Hospital between December 01, 2022 and November 30, 2023

Order	Species
Lagomorpha	Rabbit (*O cuniculus*)
Rodentia	Guinea pigs (*C porcellus*) (8.9%), chinchillas, (*C lanigera*), hamsters (Cricetinae), mouse, capybara (*H hydrochaeris*), and red and white giant flying squirrel (*Petaurista alborufus*)
Carnivora	Meerkat (*Suricata suricatta*)
Eulipotyphla	North African hedgehog (*A algirus*)
Others	Sugar glider (*P breviceps*)

Other exotic companion mammals. There were 10 ECM patients that did not belong to the major species listed above. Half (50.0%) of these were African pygmy hedgehogs (*Atelerix albiventris*), making them the most commonly presented species of other ECM, followed by 20.0% of capybaras (*Hydrochoerus hydrochaeris*). There was one case where the patient was recorded to be a member of the infraclass of Marsupialia, yet the exact species and breed of patient was not noted.

Reptiles

Thirty-three reptilian cases were presented to the NTUVH during the year, and they accounted for nearly one-fifth of all cases (18.8%). More than three-quarters (75.8%) of them were Testudines, while the remaining 24.2% were from Squamata. About 31.4% of all reptilian patients were diagnosed with gastrointestinal pathologies, while musculoskeletal problems were seen in 17.1% and skin issues were seen in 14.3% (**Table 9**).

Testudines. Gastrointestinal diseases were seen in one-third (33.3%) of all turtles and tortoises presented, while musculoskeletal disorders were diagnosed in 18.5% and pathologies of the reproductive tract was seen in 14.8%.

Chinese stripe-necked turtles (*Mauremys sinensis*) and red-eared sliders (*T scripta elegans*) were the most commonly seen turtles at NTUVH, while leopard tortoises (*Stigmochelys pardalis*) and African spurred tortoises (*Centrochelys sulcata*) were the most common species of tortoises. Each of these species accounted for 16.0% of all Testudines presented.

Squamata. Dermatologic pathologies and gastrointestinal issues were both diagnosed in 25.0% of all scaled reptiles presented. Diseases of the respiratory tract and musculoskeletal system equally shared another quarter of all cases belonging to the order of Squamata.

Scaled reptiles presented to NTUVH were mostly of the following species—the bearded dragons (*Pogona* spp), common iguanas (*Iguana iguana*), and leopard geckos (*E macularius*). Each of these species accounted for 25.0% of all Squamata cases, respectively.

Other species. There were 12 patients that did not fall into any of the major taxonomic classes and orders as listed earlier. Majority (n = 11; 91.7%) of these were cloven-hooved animals, including alpacas (*Lama pacos*) and pygmy goats, each of these species amounted to 28.5% and 21.2% of other species presented, respectively, and hence were found to be the top 2 most commonly presented species of this category.

Table 9
List of reptilian species presented at National Taiwan University Veterinary Hospital between December 01, 2022 and November 30, 2023

Order	Species
Testudines	Chinese stripe-necked turtle (*M sinensis*), diamond back terrapin (*M terrapin*), eastern painted turtle, European pond turtle (*Emys orbicularis*), and red-eared slider (*T scripta elegans*)
	Aldabra giant tortoise (*Aldabrachelys gigantea*), Greek tortoise (*Testudo graeca*), leopard tortoise (*S pardalis*), African spurred tortoise (*C sulcata*), and yellow-footed tortoise (*Chelonoidis denticulatus*)
Squamata	Bearded dragon (*Pogona* spp), common iguana (*I iguana*), leopard gecko (*E macularius*), and red-eyed crocodile skink (*Tribolonotus gracilis*)
	Corn snake (*P guttatus*)

The remaining patient that was not an ungulate was an Argentine horned frog (*Ceratophrys ornata*) presented for skin lesions (**Table 10**).

DISCUSSION
Number of Cases

The number of cases presented to CPC appeared to be 5.8 times more than that at NTUVH. The difference observed is likely caused by the variation in consultation hours of these 2 hospitals. According to the information provided from their respective official Web sites, the exotics department of CPC opens 7 days a week with its caseload shared by 2 vets[15] while that of NTUVH only opens for 3 mornings and 1 afternoon throughout a week for consultation, with all shifts equally shared among 4 vets.[16]

The number of veterinary practices and veterinarians that provide services to birds and exotic patients may have also played a role, yet to date, no official lists of veterinary clinics and/or veterinarians that offer service to nonconventional pets have were available in both countries involved in the study, hence the impact of such on case number remains unknown.

Class and Species Distribution

Overview

From the data described earlier, most commonly presented class of patients varied between the 2 hospitals. In CPC, three-quarters (75.1%) of all patients were ECM, while the most predominant class of patients seen at NTUVH were birds (37.5%). However, similarities were noted in the most common order of patients seen in each category. Members of the Psittaciformes dominated the cases of birds seen at both practices, while the order of Lagomorpha predominated the ECM presented. Similarly, turtles and tortoises were the most commonly seen reptilians.

It was worth noting that the findings of the current study did not echo with the prevalence of avian and exotic pet species previously estimated by local surveys performed in these 2 countries, respectively. According to Mercado Solutions Associates Ltd.,[11] it was deduced in Hong Kong that 25.1% of the total estimated pet population (excluding fishes) were of reptiles (14.1%), birds (6.7%), and ECM species (4.3%). Another online survey performed by Market Intelligence & Consulting

Table 10			
List of other species presented to Concordia Pet Care between December 01, 2022 and November 30, 2023 and their presumptive pathologies			
Class of Patient	Order of Patient	Patient genus/Species	Presumptive Pathologies
Mammalia	Euungulata	Alpaca (*L pacos*)	Clinically healthy
			Clinically healthy
			Open diagnosis
			Open diagnosis
		Pygmy goat	Clinically healthy
			Clinically healthy
			Open diagnosis
		Formosan sika deer (*C nippon taiouanus*)	Clinically healthy
			Clinically healthy
		Reeves's muntjac (*M reevesi*)	Clinically healthy
		Ango-nubian goat	Clinically healthy
		Donkey	Open diagnosis
Amphibia	Anura	Argentine horned frog (*C ornata*)	—

Institute[12] also estimated 39.5% of all pet owners in Taiwan owned avian and exotics species (excluding fishes), where ECM made up 17.5% of the total pet population, followed by birds (14.9%) and reptiles (7.1%).

Avian

While the most commonly presented species of birds varied between the hospitals, small-to-medium-sized parrots appeared to be the predominant type of birds seen at both services. Gastrointestinal and dermatologic pathologies were found to be 2 of the top 3 most common diagnoses seen in birds presented to these hospitals, which suggested the high prevalence of these abnormalities in birds in these countries and, hence, the need of further investigation of these common diseases in the East Asia region.

Birds seen at NTUVH were also from greater variety of order compared to that in CPC, which may also have reflected a higher acceptance toward different bird species to be kept as pets in Taiwan than in Hong Kong.

Exotic companion mammals

More than half of all ECM seen at both CPC and NTUVH were rabbits; hence, it was ranked as the most common order and species of ECM presented in both places.

Previous studies performed in the European countries have found that dental disease was the most common disease diagnosed for rabbits[1,17,18] and guinea pigs[4] presented to veterinary practices that matched with that observed in rabbits seen at NTUVH and guinea pig patients at CPC. Yet among the rabbits seen at CPC, cases diagnosed with dental disease was out-numbered by musculoskeletal pathologies, while none of the guinea pigs seen at NTUVH were diagnosed with dental issues, suggesting a different demographic prevalence of most common abnormalities in rabbits and guinea pigs in the East Asia region.

In contrast to being the second-most seen ECM species at CPC, only 2 chinchillas were presented to NTUVH, again highlight the difference in prevalence of this species among the 2 countries in the East Asia region.

Reptiles

Reptiles were ranked as the third-most presented category of patients seen at both CPC and NTUVH, with red-eared slider being the one of the most presented species in both hospitals. Such finding is coherent to that estimated in Taiwan[12] but not in Hong Kong.[11] With the mismatch in expected prevalence of pet reptiles and the clinical phenomena observed in a local exotic animal referral center, further investigation is required to examine the access to veterinary care and potentially, the overall welfare situation of these animals.

Others

While species that did not fall into the above major categories were the least presented group of patients in both hospitals involved in the study, several features were noted upon the comparison of this group of patients from CPC and NTUVH.

First, the number of cases and variety of species seen in this category was greater in NTUVH (n = 14, 9 species of animals) than that observed at CPC (n = 8, 4 species of animals). Moreover, the majority (n = 11) of these patients presented to NTUVH was cloven-footed animals, which was only the case of 1 patient seen at CPC during the analyzed timeframe. In contrast to such, more amphibians were presented to CPC (n = 4) than NTUVH (n = 1), while primates were seen at CPC but not NTUVH.

The differences observed above may be reflective of the difference in overall number and variety of species of other nonconventional pets between Hong Kong and

Taiwan, which is yet to be investigated. Another possible reason for more ungulates seen at NTUVH might be due to the fact that veterinary services for large animals were also provided under the same department ("Section of Large Animal Disease and Economic Animal Disease") as for all avian and exotic animals,[16] which was not the case for CPC in Hong Kong.

Open diagnoses

More than 10% cases seen at both hospitals (14.0% at CPC and 10.6% at NTUVH) appeared to have no confirmed diagnoses. One of the possible contributing factor may be the preference of owners when it comes to cage management, where symptomatic relief might be prioritized over the obtainment of a definitive diagnosis. Financial concerns of owners may have also played a role as suggested by a similar study performed at the University of Zurich and a recent report focusing on the trade of exotic pets in Hong Kong, as not all owners would be willing to pay the cost of specialized veterinary services that may be equivalent to or more than a few times of the monetary cost of their nonconventional pets.[1,19]

Other welfare-related observations

In addition to the similarities and differences in the situations highlighted above, some other observations were made upon reviewing and comparing the data collected.

First, a few endangered species were seen at the hospitals involved in this study, such as the critically endangered yellow-crested cockatoo (*Cacatua sulphurea*) and 2 golden coin turtles (*Cuora trifaciata*)[20] seen at CPC, and the African spurred tortoise, which was classified as an endangered species[20] was presented to both CPC and NTUVH. While the source of animal may not necessarily be the primary concern in a case management point-of-view, the existence and presentation of these animals as pets owned by members of public may be reflective of other issues faced by these species in the region, including stray and abandoned animals,[21] welfare of individuals, exotic pet trade, and poaching along with the current policies and legal enforcement of relevant regulations toward these activities.[19,22]

Moreover, Formosan sika deer (*Cervus nippon taiouanus*), Reeves's muntjac (*Muntiacus reevesi*), and Chinese stripe-necked turtles (*M sinensis*), which are native to the country were also presented to NTUVH. While it is hard to determine whether these animals were bred in captivity or obtained via another source, the suspicion of latter may get back to potential threat of poaching faced by these species.[22]

Furthermore, some groups or species of animals presented to CPC in Hong Kong have previously been reported to have inflicted injuries to their owners, namely the corn snake (*Pantherophis guttatus*), common iguana (*I iguana*), hognose snake, and turtles (Testudines).[23] Such finding reinforced the need of clear and publicly available definitions of reptilian or even exotic species suitable as pets to the general population in the country and the region of East Asia,[19] as the capability of injuring their owners have been described, while the true prevalence of such might not have been reflected in the previous study.

In addition, a few species presented to the hospitals have been reported to have established a steady local population in these countries as previously escaped pets, these included the yellow-crested cockatoos in Hong Kong,[24] common iguanas in Taiwan and red-eared sliders in both countries.[25,26] While it is uncertain if other species would follow the cases of these, such possibility should never be underestimated due to the size of the current estimated proportion of avian and exotic pets in these countries and the impact as seen in the above examples.

SUMMARY

In summary, the current study provided preliminary data on the prevalence and distribution of species presented to 2 exotics-only veterinary services in the Hong Kong and Taiwan. While this study offered a broad overview of usually encountered exotic species and their common diagnoses in 2 developed countries in the East Asia region, further studies in prevalence of species and the common diseases of nontraditional pets, along with comparison of more parameters such as age, gender, and proportion of hospitalized cases and survival rates are strongly encouraged for a greater understanding toward the current situation of avian and exotic medicine in East Asia. A longer timeframe could also be set for similar projects in the future for a better understanding toward the trends of different species and common pathologies observed over the years. Findings in these aspects would also be beneficial for all personnel working in the veterinary industry in the area to be better equipped with all skills and knowledge required for the enhancement of medical care and welfare of these animals.

CLINICS CARE POINTS

- Gastrointestinal and dermatological pathologies were found to be the most common diagnoses seen in avian patients in both Hong Kong and Taiwan, highlighting the need of further investigation in these diseases in the region.

- Rabbits are found to be the most commonly presented order and species of exotic companion mammals in the East Asia region, these patients were most often presented with musculoskeletal pathologies in Hong Kong, while dental diseases were most commonly seen in those presented in Taiwan.

- Red-eared sliders are one of the most commonly presented reptilian and testudine species in both Hong Kong and Taiwan. Those in Hong Kong were most commonly diagnosed with urinary tract and musculoskeletal disorders while those in Taiwan were mostly presented with dermatological pathologies.

- With open diagnoses seen in more than 10% cases of both hospitals involved in the study, veterinarians should be aware that further communication may be required to achieve consensus with owners towards reaching common goal(s) of case management, as well as the importance of resource allocation when financial considerations may be present.

- Veterinarians should also be more aware of the presentation of certain endangered species as privately owned animals by members of public, as such may be reflective of potential welfare-related issues in the region, such as quality of life and welfare of patient, stray and abandoned animals, poaching and exotic pet trade.

ACKNOWLEDGMENTS

The authors would like to thank Dr Zoltan Szabo, the head of Exotics Services Department of the CPC, Hong Kong and Dr Pin-Huan Yu from the Section of Large Animal Disease and Economic Animal Disease, NTUVH, Taiwan, for their permission in access, analysis, and publication of these clinical materials for this study. We are also grateful to all veterinary colleagues who worked at these 2 services for the maintenance of patient records, which served as very valuable resources for the current and future research projects. We would also like to thank those who generously provided their insights and information relevant to the design and development of this study, as the conduction of this study would not have been successful without their input. They include but not limited to the following individuals and organizations: Dr Shangzhe Xie (Mandai Wildlife Group), Dr Fiona Woodhouse (SPCA HK), Ms Vivian

Or (SPCA HK), Mr Sam Inglis (ADM Capital Foundation), Ms Christie Wong (ADM Capital Foundation), Ms Hannah Tilley (HKU), and Dr Astrid Andersson (HKU).

DISCLOSURE

The authors have nothing to disclose.

REFERENCES

1. Martin L.F., "Retrospective study on the species distribution and common diseases in exotic pets presented to the Clinic for Zoo Animals, Exotic Pets and Wildlife, University of Zurich from 2005 to 2014." University of Zurich; Switzerland. PhD diss, 2018.
2. Ángeles-Torres, Enrique Luis, Ducoing-Watty AM, et al. Identity and frequency of non-traditional companion animals presented at a university teaching hospital: a retrospective study (2009–2019). Veterinaria México OA 2023;10.
3. Nemeth NM, Gonzalez-Astudillo V, Oesterle PT, et al. A 5-year retrospective review of avian diseases diagnosed at the Department of Pathology, University of Georgia. J Comp Pathol 2016;155(2–3):105–20.
4. Minarikova A, Hauptman K, Jeklova E, et al. Diseases in pet guinea pigs: a retrospective study in 1000 animals. Vet Rec 2015;177(8):200.
5. Schmidt-Ukaj S, Hochleithner M, Richter B, et al. A survey of diseases in captive bearded dragons: a retrospective study of 529 patients. Vet Med 2017;62:9.
6. Pang VF, Pen-Heng C, Fun-In W, et al. Spontaneous neoplasms in zoo mammals, birds, and reptiles in Taiwan–a 10-year survey. Anim Biol Leiden 2012;62(no. 1): 95–110.
7. Pei-Chi H, Jane-Fang Y, Lih-Chiann W. A retrospective study of the medical status on 63 African hedgehogs (Atelerix albiventris) at the Taipei zoo from 2003 to 2011. J Exot Pet Med 2015;24(1):105–11.
8. Sheng-Chang C, Ching-Dong C, Perng-Chih S, et al. Investigation of Avian polyomavirus and Psittacine beak and Feather disease virus in parrots in Taiwan. Thai Journal of Veterinary Medicine 2021;51(2):239–45.
9. Che-Chen C, Wittawat Wechtaisong W, Shih-Yu C, et al. Prevalence and risk factors of zoonotic dermatophyte infection in pet rabbits in northern Taiwan. Journal of Fungi 2022;8(6):627.
10. Shiga T, Nakata Makoto, Miwa Yasutsugu, et al. A retrospective study (2006-2020) of cytology and biopsy findings in pet rabbits (Oryctolagus cuniculus), ferrets (Mustela putorius furo) and four-toed hedgehogs (Atelerix albiventris) seen at an exotic animal clinic in Tokyo, Japan. J Exot Pet Med 2021;38:11–7.
11. Mercado Solutions Associates Ltd. "Study on the Development of the Veterinary Profession in Hong Kong – Final Report". Agriculture, Fisheries and Conservation Department (AFCD). 2017. www.afcd.gov.hk/english/quarantine/qua_vf/files/common/VPHKFR.pdf. [Accessed 14 January 2024].
12. Market Intelligence & Consulting Institute. "【寵物消費者調查三】近七成網友曾養寵物　Z世代與未婚族是潛力飼主" www.eettaiwan.com/express/mic-2022121098 published sep 1, 2020. [Accessed January 14, 2024].
13. 三輪恭嗣. "エキゾチック動物の獣医療と今後の展望." 日本獣医師会雑誌. Journal of the Japan Veterinary Medical Association 2010;63(5):323–5.
14. American Board of Veterinary Practitioners (ABVP). "Recognised veterinary specialties, ABVP". 2023. https://abvp.com/veterinary-certification/recognized-veterinary-specialties/. [Accessed 14 January 2024].

15. Concordia Pet Care. "Concordia Pet Care: Hong Kong Pet Hospital | 24Hour Veterinary Clinic – Concordia Pet Care". en.concordiapetcare.com. [Accessed January 14, 2024].

16. National Taiwan University Veterinary Hospital. "小動物內科 - 國立臺灣大學生物資源暨農學院附設動物醫院" www.vh.ntu.edu.tw/index.php?lang=tw&do=guide&id=223 Updated Jan 8, 2024. [Accessed January 14, 2024].

17. Langenecker M, Clauss M, Hässig M, Hatt JM. "Comparative investigation on the distribution of diseases in rabbits, Guinea pigs, rats, and ferrets." Tierärztliche P. Ausgabe K. Kleintiere/Heimtiere 2009;37(5):326–33.

18. Nielsen TD, Rachel S, Dean NJ, et al. Survey of the UK veterinary profession: common species and conditions nominated by veterinarians in practice. Vet Rec 2014;174(13):324.

19. S J, Wong ETC, le Clue S, et al. Threatened, farmed: Hong Kong's invisible pets". Hong Kong SAR: ADM Capital Foundation; 2022.

20. IUCN. 'The IUCN Red List of Threatened Species. Version 2023-1'. www.iucndlist.org. [Accessed January 14, 2024].

21. Director of Bureau : Secretary for Food and Health, 2022. "Replies to initial written questions raised by Legislative Council Members in examining the Estimates of Expenditure 2022-23". Legislative Council of the Hong Kong Special Administrative Region. https://www.legco.gov.hk/yr2022/english/fc/fc/w_q/sb-e.pdf. [Accessed January 14, 2024].

22. Environmental & Animal Society of Taiwan. "台灣寵物市場販售寵物上千種！政府只管狗？動物受苦、生態遭殃、社會成本難估算！" https://www.east.org.tw/action/1492?fbclid=IwAR0kPp3lsU_EyseA461wFqjtbHsdzkTzPRj3FoOy1qDkIQGkfkgcfO1KFHk Published Sep 25, 2014. [Accessed January 14, 2024].

23. Ng Vember CH, Lit Albert CH, Wong OF, et al. Injuries and envenomation by exotic pets in Hong Kong. Hong Kong Med J 2018;24(1):48.

24. Cairns R. Poaching has decimated the numbers of this rare cockatoo. Could a feral flock in Hong Kong save the species? Cable News Network (CNN) 2023;. https://edition.cnn.com/2023/06/26/world/yellow-crested-cockatoos-hong-kong-c2e-hnk-spc-intl-scn/index.html. [Accessed 14 January 2024].

25. 陳俊宏、謝寶森、梁世雄、侯平君、邱郁文、杜銘章、吳聲海. "外來供觀賞及寵物動物之入侵研究", 國家科學委員會專題研究計畫成果報告. http://ntur.lib.ntu.edu.tw/bitstream/246246/10321/1/923114B002013.pdf Published Jul 22, 2005. [Accessed January 14, 2024].

26. Agriculture, Fisheries and Conservation Department. "Freshwater Turtle – Conservation – Threats". 2023. https://www.afcd.gov.hk/english/conservation/con_fau/con_fau_fre/con_fau_fre_con/con_fau_fre_con_thr.html. [Accessed 14 January 2024].

Exotic Animal Practice in West Asia/Middle East

Panagiotis N. Azmanis, DVM, PhD, Dip ECZM, Dip ZooMed (RCVS)[a],*,
Seyed Ahmad Madani, DVM, PhD[b], Amir Rostami, DVM, PhD[c],
Naqa Saleh Mahdi Tamimi, DVM, PhD[d],
Mark Magdy Erian, BVSc, PGDip[e]

KEYWORDS

- Middle East • West Asia • Exotics • Veterinary education • Species
- Common diseases • Ownership • Future

KEY POINTS

- Birds are the predominant taxa traditionally kept in the Middle East alongside reptiles and small mammals. Illegal trafficking and ownership of large felids, primates, reptiles, and ungulates still occur due to the lack of strict law enforcement and legislation. The primary reasons for admissions are attributed to inadequate husbandry, diet, and emergent situations.
- Exotic pet medicine is a field with scarce or virtually nonexistent university or private educational opportunities in West Asia/Middle East.
- Research remains limited, primarily encompassing epidemiologic studies focused on infectious diseases prevalent in pet shops, markets, and veterinary facilities.
- The majority of pet owners possesses limited knowledge in the realm of pet care, have restricted resources, and infrequently seek veterinary assistance.
- The provision of exotic pet medicine services predominantly occurs within mixed practices catering to small animals and exotics. Only a handful of vets in 2 countries hold board certification, prompting the local veterinary communities to express a keen interest in further advancement and progress in this field.

INTRODUCTION AND BACKGROUND OF EXOTIC ANIMAL MEDICINE IN THE MIDDLE EAST

The Middle East is a region encompassing various countries with distinct characteristics, including Turkey (Turkiye), in the north; the Levant countries (Syria, Lebanon,

[a] Dubai Falcon Hospital, 22a Street, Zabeel 2, PO BOX 23919, Dubai, United Arab Emirates;
[b] Department of Animal and Poultry Health and Nutrition, University of Tehran, Tehran, Iran;
[c] Department of Internal Medicine, University of Tehran, Tehran, Iran; [d] Department of Internal and Preventive Medicine, College of Veterinary Medicine, University of Wasit, Wasit, Iraq; [e] Department of Rafiki Vet Hospital, Cairo, Egypt
* Corresponding author. PTH10, B4 Residence Park, Dubai South, Dubai, United Arab Emirates.
E-mail address: azmanis.vet@gmail.com

Vet Clin Exot Anim 27 (2024) 521–531
https://doi.org/10.1016/j.cvex.2024.03.006
1094-9194/24/© 2024 Elsevier Inc. All rights reserved.
vetexotic.theclinics.com

Jordan, Israel, Palestine) and Egypt, in the west; the ancient Mesopotamian countries (Iraq, Kuwait), in the center; Iran, in the east; and the Persian Gulf Arab countries (Bahrain, Qatar, UAE) and the Arabian Peninsula (Kingdom of Saudi Arabia, Sultanate of Oman, Yemen), in the south. These nations differ in terms of laws, attitudes toward pet ownership, education, demographics, resources, veterinary education, and levels of care. Furthermore, the region is frequently affected by war conflicts, financial instability, and strong politics, which impede scientific exchange, cooperation, and veterinary professional development. Scientific research has primarily focused on avian infectious diseases (viral, parasitic, and bacterial) as well as dermatologic conditions in small mammals and reptiles.

TURKEY/TURKIYE(CONTRIBUTION BY D. OZGUL DVM AND K. DAYIOGLU DVM)

In Turkey, aviculture has a rich history spanning over a millennium. The Ottoman culture, deeply rooted in shamanism and reverence for nature, nurtured aviaries housing songbirds. Falconry, particularly with accipiters, also has ancient origins. Even today, public gardens in Istanbul boast aviaries. However, the ownership of exotic species and the field of exotic pet veterinary medicine are relatively new and underdeveloped. According to a recent Turkish survey conducted in 2016, 42% of the population owned small animals such as dogs and cats, 33% owned birds, 21% owned fish, 3% owned small mammals such as guinea pigs and hamsters, and 1% owned reptiles.

The education and training in exotic pet medicine provided by veterinary faculties is almost nonexistent. Only one vet school, out of the existing 32 faculties, offers a meager 1 hour elective, and there are no relevant postgraduate or continuing professional development (CPD) courses available. Teaching hospitals lack the specialized services and facilities in this field. A staggering 90% of small animal practitioners in Istanbul feel that they were not adequately trained in exotic pet medicine during their undergraduate studies.

Doves/pigeons, canaries, and other songbirds, as well as budgerigars/lovebirds, are frequently found in households. Cockatiels are not very popular, while medium-sized and large parrots remain out of reach for most people due to their expensive price. Among reptiles, the red-eared slider, iguana, bearded dragon, and native tortoise species are the most commonly kept. Small mammals such as rabbits, guinea pigs, hamsters, and rats also enjoy popularity. According to a survey conducted among small animal practices in Istanbul, avian species make up 42.4% of the presented exotic pets, followed by chelonians at 32%, other reptiles at 16.9%, and fish at 8.4%.

Common diseases that afflict exotic pets are linked to inadequate diet and husbandry practices. Exotic small mammals often suffer from dental and gastrointestinal issues, as well as ovarian cysts and various dermatologic conditions. Reptiles commonly grapple with metabolic bone disease (MBD). Birds, apart from issues related to their diet and husbandry, are admitted for orthopedic, dermatologic, respiratory, and traumatic etiologies.

The financial constraints faced by low-income individuals who keep small aviary birds often hinder their ability to seek veterinary care or afford diagnostic tests. The expense associated with ectoparasite treatment or vaccination for small mammals is perceived as exorbitant by some. Unfortunately, a significant number of pet owners possess a mindset that undervalues the importance of their pets' well-being, resulting in negligence toward their health. However, there are bird owners who uphold family traditions and prioritize addressing health issues and providing proper care for their feathered companions. It is worth noting that the majority of reptile owners lack proper education, leading to a sad statistical where approximately 90% of imported iguanas fail to survive until adulthood. Those that do survive often suffer from MBD and overall poor health. Among the few educated clients who seek the expertise of an exotic veterinarian, only a small percentage of clients are willing to bear the expenses associated with diagnosis and treatment.

Regarding private practice and future prospects, owners typically turn first to pet shops and traders for advice. There are no board-certified exotic veterinarians and experienced professionals in the field. Small animal clinics provide all exotic animal services. In Istanbul, exotic pets account for merely 1% to 10% of the caseload in 91.4% of small animal practices. A recent study conducted among small animal practitioners in Istanbul revealed that 53% of them had limited familiarity with exotic pet diseases. Additionally, 65% felt confident in their knowledge of avian medicine but acknowledged a lack of expertise in reptilian and fish medicine.[1] Despite many veterinarians claiming to practice exotic pet medicine or expressing an interest in it, they often lack the necessary knowledge and skills, leading to dissatisfaction among pet owners. Furthermore, veterinarians tend to be reluctant to invest in CPD in exotic animal medicine, as they do not perceive it to be financially lucrative.

LEVANT COUNTRIES (SYRIA, LEBANON, JORDAN, ISRAEL, AND PALESTINE)

The information available for these countries is quite limited. In Syria, there are 4 veterinary faculties in Hama, Al-Forat, Aleppo, and Damascus universities. There is no special course dedicated to exotic pets for veterinary students in these universities and there is no postgraduate or residency program for exotic pet medicine in Syria. Pet birds such as canaries, other small passerines, and pigeons are the most popular exotic animals in Syria. Private clinics are growing in number in recent years especially in big cities such as Damascus, but continuing educations and training programs are rare if any (Contributed by F. Almasri, BVSc, PhD; Damascus University).

In Lebanon, the Veterinary Department of the Agronomy Faculty at the Lebanese University offers a 16 hour specialized course in new companion animals (exotics) during the final year of study. Only a few small animal practices that provide basic care for exotics.

In Jordan, there is only one veterinary faculty that provides a 1 hour electronic undergraduate course on exotic and marine animal medicine, but unfortunately, there are no postgraduate courses available. The teaching hospital does not have a specialized service for exotic pets. However, it is interesting to observe that the ownership of exotic animals has increased, particularly following the COVID pandemic. Jordanian owners have a diverse range of exotics, including fish, parrots, and tortoises.

In Israel, up until 2005, the number of clinics and veterinarians specializing in exotics was extremely limited. The Koret Veterinary Faculty of the Hebrew University offered its students a 3 credit avian/exotic course during their second year of study. The curriculum also included courses on poultry, fish, and bee medicine. From 2005 and onward, an advanced course (elective) was introduced for third year students. After 2008, the original syllabus began to shrink. The basic course was then reduced to a mere 2 credits, which is truly insufficient. From 2010 to 2011, there was no longer an exotic service at the Veterinary Teaching Hospital (VTH), and a reduced course was taught by volunteers, none of whom held any board certification. The situation remains the same until present. Over the past 2 decades, there has been a remarkable increase of rabbit ownership, positioning them as the third most popular companion animals, trailing behind dogs and cats. In a bustling exotic veterinary clinic, it is estimated that approximately 60% of the caseload is composed of pet rabbits, a stark contrast to 20 years ago when parrots prevailed. Pet birds still hold a significant presence with multiple breeders and private individuals keeping a variety of avian species, ranging from budgerigar to hyacinth macaw. Alongside rabbits, there has also been an increase in other small mammals such as guinea pigs, rats, ferrets, and sugar gliders. The most prevalent reptilian species include the green iguana, corn snake, ball python, leopard gecko, and various tortoise species. Dental issues, spaying and neutering procedures, purchase health checks, nail trimming, sarcoptic mange, and urolithiasis are all common afflictions in rabbits and other exotic mammals. Feather picking, various infections, and heavy metal intoxication are common presentations in parrots. Reptiles experience conditions such as MBD, egg binding, burns, and pneumonia. In recent years, the proliferation of purebred rabbits, Facebook communities, and breeders has contributed to the expansion of the exotic market. Reptile owners often opt for self-medication and advice from pet shops and friends rather than seeking professional veterinary assistance. Israeli pet owners could be considered equally educated to the North American counterparts, due to the widespread availability of information on the Internet, coupled with the prevalent English proficiency among the Israeli population (contributed by A. Gancz DVM, DVSc, Dip European College of Zoological Medicine [ECZM]).

In West Bank of Palestine in An-Najah National University, there is undergraduate course of rabbit production and diseases, but no undergraduate or postgraduate course on exotic pet medicine. Pet ownership has been growing in West Bank and Gaza Strip in recent years, and few private veterinary clinics have been opened for companion animal veterinary services.

EGYPT

Traditionally, Egyptians have maintained a diverse array of avian companions, including pigeons (for various purposes), songbirds, and budgerigars. However, in the past 5 years, there has been a noticeable surge in the popularity of medium and large parrots for both keeping and breeding. Smaller psittacine birds such as budgerigars, lovebirds, and cockatiels are typically regarded as aviary birds and are not commonly kept as in-house pets.

In Egypt, there are a total of 16 veterinary faculties, but only 4 of them offer a syllabus dedicated to the study of small companion animals (specifically dogs and cats). Unfortunately, there is currently no syllabus available for the field of exotic animal medicine. However, 2 veterinary faculties do boast a dedicated Wildlife/Zoo Medicine Department, along with a theoretic postgraduate course in pathology and zoo medicine. The few veterinarians practicing exotic animal medicine (∼10–15 professionals) are primarily self-taught with limited opportunities for CPD.

Among the most popular medium and large parrot species kept in Egypt are the gray parrot, Alexandrine parakeet, and Indian ring-necked parakeet. In recent years, there has also been successful breeding of macaws. The Egyptian tortoise, along with other native tortoise species such as the Greek tortoise and Hermann's tortoise, are the second commonly kept pets. Remarkably, it is estimated that 1 in every 20 households in Egypt has a tortoise. As for mammalian pets, guinea pigs and hamsters top the list of commonly kept species. Rabbits are predominantly raised for meat production purposes. Additionally, vervet monkeys are frequently kept as pets and subsequently presented to veterinarians for their care. Notably, the vast majority of reptiles and monkeys are illegally owned and obtained through animal trafficking trade.

Common diseases in exotic pets encompass a range of health concerns, including respiratory infections, intestinal parasitism, dehydration/gout, feather destructive behavior, enteritis, and bacterial respiratory infections caused by *Klebsiella sp, Pseudomonas sp, and Proteus sp*. Additionally, dietary problems such as hepatic lipidosis, vitamin deficiency, hypocalcemia/secondary hyperparathyroidism, gastrointestinal stasis, and dental issues (such as elongation, uneven wore pattern, and abscess) may arise in guinea pigs and rabbits due to inadequate diet. Trauma, respiratory infection, and hypocalcemia are also prevalent in vervet monkeys as a result of chronic poor diet. Parrot owners commonly seek advice from pet stores and breeders rather than consulting veterinarians. In a busy veterinary practice, approximately 30% to 50% of the caseload is composed of exotic pets, while the remaining are dogs and cats. The breeding of parrots has witnessed a significant surge in the past 5 years, with hobby breeders estimated to produce around 20,000 parrots annually. The regulation of exotic pet ownership pertains solely to matters of importation and travel. Smuggling of exotics is a frequent occurrence, often taking place through the Sudan borders in the south, the Sinai/Negev desert in the east, and the Libyan desert in the west. The small falconry community visits infrequently a veterinarian.

IRAQ

Currently, there is a notable absence of scientific training or educational opportunities in Iraq for exotic pet medicine. This deficiency extends to all 8 veterinary faculties, leaving veterinarians unprepared to effectively deal with exotic animals and wildlife. Consequently, veterinary clinics rarely receive exotic animals, and pet owners are left to rely on self-education to meet their pets' needs. Aviculture is an exception to this trend. Fresh graduate veterinarians gain practical experience in pet medicine by working alongside experienced senior doctors. Scientific research on exotic animals in Iraq is limited, primarily focusing on rabbits, guinea pigs, and turtles. Birds have received comparatively more attention due to their diverse nature and people's interest in keeping them as pets.

Birds are the most prevalent types of exotic pets in Iraq. Racing pigeons, parrots, canaries, finches, turkeys, raptors, and various other bird species have been kept by Iraqis as pets or housed in aviaries. On the other hand, reptiles are less popular as pets in Iraq, with people showing greater preference for birds, cats, and dogs. This preference arises from the challenges associated with reptile care and the traditional fear surrounding this taxon. Furthermore, various apes, deer, guinea pigs, hamsters, rabbits, squirrels, and hedgehogs are kept. There is still a trend to keep wildlife species such as lions, wolves, jaguars, tigers (including white variants), and cheetahs. Tortoises and turtles are the most common reptiles in Iraq alongside fewer snakes, geckos, green iguanas, bearded dragons, monitor lizards, and caimans.

The ownership of exotic pets in Iraq can be considered low, limited to a select group of passionate individuals who possess the means to acquire an exotic species. Although the exact number of these individuals remains unrecorded, it is estimated to be quite small. Interestingly, bird owners constitute the largest segment among all pet owners, numbering some hundreds of thousands, if not more. Iraqis show an increasing preference to either keep birds in cages within their homes or allow them to freely roam indoors. Aviculture gains also significant popularity. The relatively low cost of wild animals, such as lions, priced as low as 3000 dollars, proves tempting for novice owners. Consequently, various types of animals are imported, smuggled, or unlawfully obtained from nature, finding their way into the hands of these passionate individuals across the country, with little to no regulations in place to control or organize such practices. In the absence of specialized veterinarians, passionate owners have formed groups to exchange essential information regarding the proper care and treatment. Reptiles-IQ stands as an example.

The majority of health issues affecting exotic and wild animals can be attributed to improper husbandry and inadequate nutrition. Large felids are often diagnosed with MBD and parvovirus infection in unvaccinated cubs. Furthermore, external parasites, such as lice, fleas, and ticks and dermatologic fungal infections have been diagnosed. In guinea pigs, urolithiasis and root elongation are the most prevalent health concerns, while respiratory problems and snake mites pose significant challenges for reptiles. MBD and root elongation are the leading health issues among rabbits. Commercial diets catering to nearly all species of birds are readily available throughout the country. However, the options for hamsters, guinea pigs, rabbits, and turtles remain relatively limited, with only a few brands to choose from. Many reptile owners breed small mammals to provide to their reptiles, while mealworms are readily available in pet shops as bird food.

The current number of exotic pet owners is relatively low (except for birds); nevertheless, a few young owners are pioneering to create pages and accounts on various social media platforms, propagating exotic pet ownership. A potential increase in the number of exotic pet enthusiasts could be anticipated in the near future. The Faculty of Veterinary Medicine at the University of Baghdad intends to include exotic pet medicine in the future curriculum for students.

IRAN

The Assyrian relief found in the Khorsaad ruins in Iraq, dating back to 1700 BC stands as a remarkable testament to the earliest depiction of falconry in human history. These ancient murals at Persepolis, dating back to 500 BC, also portray wild and exotic animals, including lions, okapis, and deer, which were presented as gifts to the Persian king. The literature of ancient Persia, particularly the Masnavi written by the renowned poet Jalal al-Din Muhammad Balkhi (1207–1273), provides extensive documentation on the importation and domestication of exotic psittacine species such as the ring-necked parakeet and Alexandrine parakeet for keeping as pet birds. Moreover, historical Persian poems and folkloric stories shed light on the oldest caged passerine birds in Iran, namely the common nightingales (*Luscinia megarhynchos*) and white-eared bulbuls (*Pycnonotus leucotis*). Despite the tradition of keeping wild animals by Persian kings was deeply rooted in Iranian history, it was during the Qajar dynasty (1789–1925) that the keeping of various exotic animals by ordinary people was documented.

The inception of the first modern school for veterinary medicine education in Iran dates back to 1932, known as Madreseyeh-Alie-Beitari (the Higher Education School for Veterinary Medicine). At present, Iran has 25 veterinary schools. Recognizing the paramount significance of training veterinarians in exotic animal diseases, the subject of exotic animal diseases was successfully incorporated into the Doctor of Veterinary Medicine (DVM) and postgraduate curriculum at the Faculty of Veterinary Medicine, University of Tehran, commencing in 2001. Prior to 2005, there was no dedicated course syllabus focused on exotic birds and pet avian medicine. A segment from the poultry course was allocated to cover these subjects. Starting from 2009, the practical rotation course syllabus in avian medicine was expanded, providing a training opportunity for Iranian veterinary students. Furthermore, an elective course in avian medicine, spanning 2 hours per week, was introduced into the DVM course syllabus in 2017. Now, there are no postgraduate academic programs or residencies in Iran specializing solely in avian/exotic pet medicine. Instead, the discipline of companion and exotic avian medicine is encompassed within the poultry disease specialty, which is a postgraduate combined course/thesis-based academic program with a history spanning over 3 decades in Iranian universities. This comprehensive program encompasses various aspects of avian medicine, such as avian anesthesia and surgery, diseases of pet birds, diseases of wild birds, and diagnostic imaging in avian medicine. Postgraduate students, referred to as poultry residents, undergo 4 semesters of coursework and clinical rotations at the university avian clinic. Upon successful completion, they become eligible to take the specialty board examination. Successful candidates are also required to conduct research for their thesis and defend it, thereby earning a postgraduate doctorate degree specializing in the field of avian diseases. While research theses predominantly focused on poultry diseases until 2009, subsequent research projects have included pet avian diseases. In 2013, the inception of the first specialized pet bird clinic within the Faculty of Veterinary Medicine at the University of Tehran marked a significant milestone. Prior to this, clinical services were offered in the same clinic as commercial poultry. The new clinic is now situated within the small animal teaching hospital. In recent years, the country has witnessed exponential growth in the number of specialized veterinary clinics and hospitals, with a minimum of 5 private avian exclusively vet practices in Tehran alone. Continuing education in the field of avian medicine has been ardently pursued by the Iran Veterinary Council since 2011, with workshops, wet laboratories, and online courses offered annually for veterinarians. Moreover, a multitude of research projects on exotic pets have been undertaken as student theses, culminating in the publication of scientific articles in esteemed international journals. Over the past decade, educational workshops focusing on exotic animal diseases have also been organized to educate private practitioners throughout Iran.

The ownership of exotic pets has a long-standing tradition in Iran, and there has been a notable increase in recent years. Iranians keep various exotic animals, including small mammals and reptiles. In a statistical study conducted from 2021 to 2023, a total of 2390 exotic pets were examined at the Teaching Hospital of the Faculty of Veterinary Medicine at the University of Tehran. Among these, approximately 65% were rabbits, 15% were guinea pigs, 5% were small mammals (such as hamsters, Persian squirrels, and hedgehogs), and 15% were reptiles (including tortoises, terrapins, lizards, and snakes). A census conducted by the Statistical Center of Iran in 2003 revealed that the country had a population of 24,783,000 backyard chickens and 5,916,000 other backyard poultry, such as turkeys, ducks, and geese. Although commercial poultry production has witnessed significant growth in the past 2 decades, the population of backyard poultry appears to have remained unchanged since the previous census. Estimating the number of other pet and exotic birds is a challenging task, if not an impossible one. In Iran, birds pose as the most favored companion animals, due to religious and cultural customs. In contrast to certain Arabian countries, falconry is not a popular practice in Iran. In fact, it is strictly prohibited due to species conservation. The most commonly owned and presented cage birds in Iran are Psittaciformes (75% of avian cases) and Passeriformes (11%).

"The Office of Animal Disease Control and Serum Production" was primarily founded in 1925. This office was promoted to the Iran Veterinary Organization (IVO) by national parliament legislation in 1971. Prevention and control of all animal diseases, including zoo, wild, and exotic animals, are legal duties of the IVO. The hunting and fishing laws were legislated in 1967 for protecting wild and exotic animals in Iran. In 1971, Iran hosted the Ramsar Convention on Wetlands of International Importance. After its institution in 1971, the Department of Environment in Iran oversees the breeding, importing, and exporting of nondomestic animals, including exotic pet species. Iran has been a member of the Convention on International Trade in Endangered

Species of Wild Fauna and Flora (CITES) since 1976. Therefore, CITES regulations on the trade of exotic animals are in place and practiced in the country. According to the enactments by the Supreme Environment Council, the wild animals of Iran are further classified as endangered, protected, not protected, and invasive pests. The capture and ownership of all endangered and protected species are illegal. Nevertheless, illegal smuggling of exotic birds from the eastern borders is still the main route of entry for exotic psittacine birds. In addition to the CITES approval issued by the Department of Environment, a health certificate from the national veterinary authorities is required for any trade of exotic species. Health requirements for the import of different species are regulated by the IVO. The minimum requirement for all avian species is the absence of notifiable infectious diseases such as avian influenza and Newcastle disease. Although cockfighting is illegal, there are reports of covert contests taking place in certain provinces.

Just like in other parts of the world, pet bird owners and clients can be classified into 4 distinct categories. The first group comprises naïve/new owners who have recently acquired a bird but are not yet familiar with their biology. The second category comprises experienced aviculturists who engage in hobby breeding and are familiar with their pets' routines and behaviors. The third group comprises experienced professionals, including bird fanciers, pet breeders, and zoo and aviary keepers (eg, canary owners, backyard and free-range poultry farmers, pigeon fanciers). The last group of clients are the inexperienced owners who illusion a sense of knowledge. This group includes many owners of small passerines, pigeon fanciers, illegal cockfighting enthusiasts, and even some pet shop employees. Common pitfalls encountered with this group involve improper ownership practices, misuse of medication, unnecessary prescription of antibiotics, and failure to adhere to veterinary instructions. In recent years, the Faculty of Veterinary Medicine at the University of Tehran, along with various hospitals in Tehran, has organized workshops aimed at educating owners on the proper care and management of different species of mammals and reptiles. Even during the COVID-19 outbreak, these workshops have successfully transitioned to virtual platforms.

Common diseases in exotic pets encompass a range of health issues, including problems associated with husbandry malpractices, malnutrition, traumatic lesions, and poor owner–pet interaction. Psittacine birds, specifically, are prone hypovitaminosis A and calcium deficiency. Additionally, gastrointestinal dysbiosis is a common occurrence in young pet birds. Iron storage disease is prevalent among captive common mynahs (*Acridotheres tristis*). Trichomoniasis is the most prevalent protozoal infection in pet birds in Iran, especially in pigeons, common mynahs, and other passerines. A novel *Isospora* sp has been documented in common mynahs. Notably, various metazoan parasites have been reported in exotic birds such as tracheal mites (*Ptilonyssus morofskyi*) affecting canaries and air sac nematodiasis (*Diplotriaena* sp) as respiratory parasites in common mynahs. Fungal diseases, such as aspergillosis, candidiasis, and macrorhabdosis, are frequently encountered in avian practice in Iran. Antemortem diagnosis mainly relies on mycological investigation, cytologic findings, and diagnostic imaging. Radiology and ultrasonography are routinely employed in exotic pet practice across various teaching hospitals and private clinics. Computed tomography is exclusively accessible at the small animal teaching hospital of the University of Tehran. Additionally, 2 private hospitals in Tehran have recently acquired MRI machines. Laparoscopy and endoscopy procedures are performed in selected veterinary teaching hospitals, private hospitals, or clinics. Soft tissue and orthopedic surgeries are commonly carried out in numerous clinics, with isoflurane anesthesia machines readily available in a multitude of academic and private clinics. Similarly, exotic mammals and reptiles are admitted for husbandry, nutrition, and metabolic diseases. Malocclusion and root elongation are frequently observed in rabbits and guinea pigs, while MBD is prevalent in squirrels and various reptile species. Terrapins often suffer from hypovitaminosis A, while reptiles commonly face gout-related issues. In more detail, rabbit clostridial enteropathy is the most common bacterial complication, while coccidiosis, *Encephalitozoon cuniculi*, and skin parasites such as *Sarcoptes scabiei* are the most significant parasitic infections. Guinea pigs may also experience lice infestations caused by *Gliricidia porcelli*, in addition to clostridial enteropathy. In hamsters, older female hamsters are typically referred due to pyometra, which involves bacterial agents such as *Streptobacillus moniliformis, Escherichia coli, and Arcanobacterium pyogenes* followed by atrial thrombosis. Squirrels, apart from MBD, are frequently plagued by external parasites, such as the louse *Neohaematopinus sp.* Reptiles commonly suffer from salmonellosis and its complications, considering its zoonotic significance. Owners are provided with necessary training to prevent disease transmission. Although recent studies have been conducted on *Chlamydia* and herpes virus infections in pet reptiles, no positive results have been obtained thus far. In a study on parasitic infections in pet reptiles, protozoa and nematodes were found in 52% of the cases. The identified protozoans include *Trichomonads, Balantidium, Cryptosporidium, Isospora, Eimeria,* and *Amebae.* Additionally, cases of dermatophytosis caused by *Trichophyton mentagrophytes* have been reported in pet reptiles.

Iranian veterinarians possess the expertise to handle various clinical scenarios with utmost competence. Over the last few decades, intricate networks based on cooperation and knowledge have been established, largely due to the advancement of diverse social network platforms. Undoubtedly, the exotic pet practice will experience exponential improvement in the years to come. The establishment of residency and academic programs in this domain is an urgent necessity that will undoubtedly be introduced in due course. International collaboration is both a current and future prerequisite for veterinary practice in Iran. The most significant impediment to the qualitative advancement of exotic pet practice in Iran lies in the economic constraints and sanctions, which impede access to state-of-the-art medical equipment.

ARAB STATES OF THE PERSIAN GULF AND ARABIAN PENINSULA (KUWAIT, BAHRAIN, QATAR, UNITED ARAB EMIRATES, OMAN, SAUDI ARABIA, AND YEMEN)

The most emblematic species kept over 4000 years is the falcon (saker, peregrine, and Barbary) as part of the United Nations Educational, Scientific and Cultural Organization (UNESCO)-protected falconry tradition. Interestingly, despite being neighboring countries, Yemen and Oman do not have a falconry tradition. In recent years, there has been a noticeable increase in the keeping of pets, including exotics, influenced by Western expats residing in these countries. Wealthy individuals in the past used to keep a wide range of exotic animals as pets, such as primates, large felids, hyenas, slow lorises, owls, various species of ungulates, crocodiles, and poisonous reptiles.[2,3] However, in the UAE, the practice of keeping such animals has become more restricted due to the implementation of the Federal Law on Dangerous Animals (2016). This law criminalizes the keeping of dangerous animals as pets, and offenders may face fines ranging from 10,000 to 500,000 Dhs (2500–125,000 USD). Additionally, the UAE CITES office now meticulously scrutinizes every case of animal import/export to and from the UAE. Oman has also strict laws on wildlife conservation and trade.

Education and training in exotic pet medicine is limited and some of the smaller emirates such as Bahrain, Kuwait, and Qatar do not have a veterinary faculty. Similarly, the Kingdom of Saudi Arabia and the Sultanate of Oman currently lack a syllabus for exotic pet medicine. The UAE University stands out as it offers a syllabus dedicated to exotic pet medicine through its Department of Veterinary Medicine.

A significant development in providing high-quality accredited veterinary education, specifically in small animal, equine, and exotic pet medicine, was the launch of the Middle East African Veterinary Conference in 2022. This conference, which will continue in 2024, aims to provide CPD and has received accreditation from the American Association of Veterinary State Boards Registry of Approved Continuing Education approval and the Veterinary Continuing Education in Europe. Over the past 5 years, there has also been an avian symposium focused on avian and zoo practitioners. This symposium, sponsored by a local pharmaceutical veterinary company, offers CPD opportunities, including lectures by international and local speakers, as well as wet laboratories. However, this symposium is not accredited. In the past, an international conference on falcon/raptor medicine was held in Qatar but has since been discontinued.

Over the past 8 to 10 years, the exotic pet trade has witnessed a substantial growth due to the emergence of improved animal markets and pet stores that offer a wide range of species. These species include parrots, toucans, songbirds, finches, mynahs, ratites, reptiles, rabbits, guinea pigs, African hedgehogs, sugar gliders, and hamsters. Furthermore, there is an active community of fish enthusiasts and aquarists, as well as pigeon enthusiasts who breed and showcase pigeons.

Avian patients are often brought in for initial health assessments, issues related to inadequate diet, feather-plucking behavior, traumas, and emaciation. Small mammals typically require initial health assessments, vaccinations, castration/neutering, dental and gastrointestinal pathology, and treatment of skin diseases. Reptiles commonly suffer from MBD, burn wounds, stomatitis, mites, and respiratory disease.

Within the avian community, there are numerous knowledgeable owners, including falconers, parrot owners, and pigeon enthusiasts. These owners possess adequate knowledge and experience not only in the care and diet but also in the prevention and treatment of diseases. There are numerous Web sites and Facebook groups dedicated to tortoises, pigeons, parrots, and other species. Additionally, there are owner groups of trained parrots advocating free-flying or flying on a leash as well as experienced avian trainers who participate in zoo shows and private events. While the majority of owners, particularly western expatriates, are attentive and willing to invest in their pets' wellness, there are still many uninformed owners who impulsively acquire parrots or reptiles and provide inadequate diets and care. These owners typically seek veterinary assistance only when their pet's condition becomes critical, often resulting in chronic issues. Many parrots are mistakenly fed chick formula for months, as instructed by the pet store, and fail to properly transition to a suitable diet. Consequently, a significant number of parrots and reptiles fail to reach maturity and succumb to premature death.

Currently, there exist 1 ECZM (avian)/RCVS ZooMed specialist and a total of 4 American College of Zoological Medicine (ACZM) board-certified practitioners. Additionally, there are a few Royal College of Veterinary Surgeons (RCVS) CertZooMed holders, practicing in private practice. In the majority of countries, the availability of board-certified veterinarians is limited, resulting in exotic animal services being typically provided by mixed small animal practices or clinics. The Gulf countries boast approximately 20 falcon clinics/hospitals, both governmental and private, that adhere to a commendable standard of avian practice. Some for-profit falcon hospitals have expanded their range of services to include other avian species and exotic animals. Furthermore, there has been a surge in the establishment of avian/exotic animal practices over the past 5 years. Consequently, many small animal clinics now have an avian/exotic animal practitioner as part of their staff. In Oman and Saudi Arabia, only few practices offer basic exotic pet medicine, while currently there are no data for Yemen.

Summarizing, in West Asia/Middle East region, birds were and still are the commonest exotic pet kept, especially as aviary or falconry birds. Undergraduate and postgraduate education courses are absent and demanded by modern mixed practitioners (small animals/exotics). Other pet species are also on the rise, while sadly still illegal trafficking of primates, large felids, and other animals is still practiced. The vets are faced with the universal husbandry/diet-related medical problems in birds, reptiles, and small mammals. Avian/falconry medicine is a well-advanced field in the countries that falconry is practiced, benefiting as well other exotic pet species. Finally, research is basic and involves universities and epidemiology of viral and parasitic pathogens.

REFERENCES

1. SIĞIRCI BD, Serkan İKİZ, Celik B, et al. A survey study on self-evaluations of small pet practitioners about exotic pets in Istanbul in 2016. Acta Veterinaria Eurasia 2019;45(1):9–15.
2. Spee LB, Hazel SJ, Dal Grande E, et al. Endangered exotic pets on social media in the Middle East: Presence and impact. Animals 2019;9(8):480.
3. Tamimi NS, Bahare T, Shahram J, et al. A retrospective study on 1587 exotic pets presented to the small animal veterinary hospital, University of Tehran. Iraqi Journal of Veterinary Medicine 2020;44(E0):1–6.

Exotic Animal Practice in Southeast Asia

Rina Maguire, BVSc hons 1, Dipl ABVP Exotic Companion Mammals, Dipl
ACEPM[b],*, Qianying Athena Lim, BSc, BVMS[b],
Ali Anwar Bin Ahmad, DVM (UPM), Dipl ACCM, CertAqV[a]

KEYWORDS

- ASEAN exotic pet health care • Exotic pet medical development • SEA

KEY POINTS

- The animal health industry in Southeast Asia (SEA) has experienced increased growth in the last 30 years, and it looks set to continue growing at pace.
- In our survey of veterinary practices, exotic pets presented mainly for illnesses (55%) as well as preventive wellness examinations (35%) and emergencies (9%).
- Exotic practitioners have access to standard or modified veterinary and human equipment including in-house clinical pathology (83%), radiology (73%), ultrasound (63%), and advanced imaging (13%).
- Veterinary interest organizations for exotic animals in several SEA countries have successfully built an interest in this emerging field by sharing knowledge in continuing education events, providing a platform for discussing cases, and pushing for the inclusion of exotic pet health in veterinary undergraduate programs.

INTRODUCTION

Over the past several decades, the pet industry has seen a surge of interest in exotic animal ownership, and the demand for exotic animal pet health care has risen in many Southeast Asia (SEA) countries Appendix 1–3. This region consists of 11 countries including Brunei, Cambodia, Indonesia, Laos, Malaysia, Myanmar, Philippines, Singapore, Thailand, Timor Leste, and Vietnam. SEA has among the world's highest biodiversity.[1] Wild animals in the region are traded extensively for the exotic pet market.[2] In the last 3 decades, there has been geopolitical peace and a robust economy, which has seen SEA rise as a great economic power.[3,4] In addition to the more conventional exotic animal pets, SEA faces a dilemma with less restricted trading of

[a] Veterinary Healthcare, Mandai Wildlife Group, 80 Mandai Lake Road, Singapore 729826;
[b] Avian and Exotics, Beecroft Animal Specialist & Emergency Hospital, 991E Alexandra Road, #01-27, Singapore 119973
* Corresponding author.
E-mail address: rina.maguire@birdvet.com.sg

Vet Clin Exot Anim 27 (2024) 533–549
https://doi.org/10.1016/j.cvex.2024.03.007
1094-9194/24/© 2024 Elsevier Inc. All rights reserved.

vetexotic.theclinics.com

wildlife species destined as pets. As one of the global hubs of illegal wildlife trading, trading of wildlife occurs in local marketplaces and online in many SEA countries.[5] Despite increased legislation in many SEA countries to curb the illegal wildlife trade, the enforcement of these laws in most of these countries is still an ongoing source of frustration.

Veterinary care standards for exotic animals in SEA have traditionally been slower to reach what is considered the gold standard. Education of the public to provide good health care for exotic animals can be challenging due to the perceived low value of the pet and the high cost of veterinary services. Many vets face challenges in receiving training in this field due to the lack of continuing education opportunities and training available locally. Undergraduate veterinary degrees in SEA have a focus on agriculture, livestock management, and large animal medicine. This is because all the SEA countries except Singapore and Brunei, still thrive on agriculture as the main economic driving force. These 2 countries are the only exceptions to having a university offering a veterinary degree. Students from these countries interested in becoming veterinarians would have to study abroad before getting licensure in their home countries.

In recent years, there has been a steady improvement in the educational opportunities and support for veterinarians interested in this field. This has led to promising changes and greater opportunities for a career as a clinician working with exotic pet animals in SEA. This article presents the results of a survey of exotic animal clinicians in different countries in SEA including Singapore, Malaysia, Indonesia, the Philippines, and Thailand to describe the exotic animal practices in different countries. We also interviewed veterinary associations in the region with an interest in wildlife and exotic medicine and leaders in the field to get historical information on how exotic medicine developed and ongoing programs geared to promote exotic medicine. The interviewees were also asked about the future trajectory of the exotic field in their respective countries. We hope that this knowledge will help future efforts in improving the landscape of exotic animal medicine in SEA (**Fig. 1**).

CURRENT EVIDENCE

Information regarding the exotic medicine practice in SEA was collected from an online survey that was emailed to veterinary clinics in SEA promoted as exotic practices. The responses from the survey were collected between August and December 2023. Only one response from a veterinarian who treats exotics was accepted from each clinic. The online survey was generated in Google Form, and it consists of a series of short answer and multiple-choice questions. The questions focused on the type of exotics practice (exotics only or mixed small animals/exotics), type of species seen, reasons for presentation, availability of veterinary referrals, and access to in-house clinical pathology (cytology, serum biochemistry, hematology, fecal analysis, and urinalysis), diagnostic imaging such as radiography and ultrasounds, endoscopy, and advanced imaging (computed tomography and MRI) when treating exotic animals. A total of 30 responses were received from veterinary clinics in Singapore, Malaysia, Indonesia, Thailand, the Philippines, and Brunei. No responses were received from Laos, Vietnam, and Cambodia. No invitation to the survey was sent to Timor Leste and Myanmar due to the inability to find relevant exotic practices in these 2 countries. The number of responses varied with each country. The responses to the survey for the SEA countries are Malaysia 53.3% (n = 16), Singapore 20% (n = 6), followed by Thailand 6.7% (n = 2), Indonesia 6.7% (n = 2), Brunei 3.3% (n = 1), and Philippines 10% (n = 3) (Appendix 1). Exotic species seen in SEA clinics

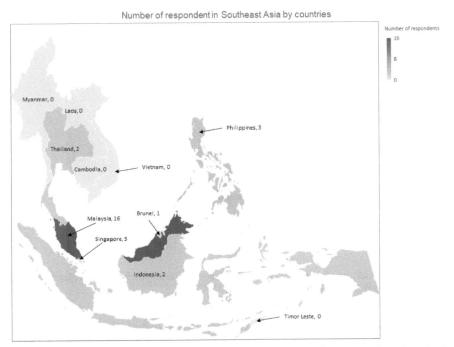

Fig. 1. The geographic distribution of the respondents in SEA to the survey of exotic animal practice performed in this study.

include avian species, exotic small mammals, reptiles, amphibians, large felines, and primates. Most respondents (27 out of 30) work in practices that treat canine, feline, and exotic animal species. Exotic pets presented to vet practices across SEA were categorized into emergencies, illnesses, and general wellness consultations (**Fig. 2**). On average, emergency presentations are highest in Singapore, with 25% of cases being emergencies. Exotics practices surveyed in the Philippines and Brunei have the highest cases seen for illnesses: 70% and 100%, respectively. The 2 exotic clinics in Indonesia reported the highest numbers of wellness examinations for exotic patients in SEA with 70% of the overall cases classified as wellness. There are only 3 exotics-exclusive practices in SEA, which are located in the major cities of Kuala Lumpur in Malaysia, Singapore, and Bangkok in Thailand. The practices in Thailand and Malaysia are standalone exotic facilities. The exotics specialist referral practice in Singapore is located within a 24 hour emergency hospital facility with other referral specialists' services. Surgeries conducted on exotic patients are categorized into orthopedics, elective soft tissue, and nonelective soft tissue procedures. The elective cases would include nonemergency surgeries such as castration, spaying, and dermal mass removals. Nonelective cases conducted would include laparotomies, surgical correction, eye surgeries, dental procedures, urolith removals, shell repairs, egg extractions for egg binding, and wound repairs. **Fig. 3** shows procedures conducted in SEA's practices that responded to the survey. Malaysia shows the highest number of clinics that conduct elective (9), nonelective (12), and orthopedic (4) procedures in SEA.

The diagnostic capabilities to treat exotics appear to be readily available (Appendix 2). In the survey, 83% of the respondents from Malaysia, Thailand, Philippines, Singapore,

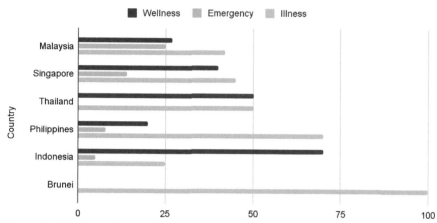

Fig. 2. Classification of exotic animal consultations divided into 3 types (wellness, emergency, and illness) in exotic animal practices in SEA.

Indonesia, and Brunei have access to in-house clinical pathology. Radiography was available in 73% and ultrasound services are available in 63% of clinics surveyed. There are 4 practices (13%) with access to advanced imaging including 1 practice in the Philippines, 1 in Thailand, and 2 practices in Singapore. The hospital in Singapore has access to a 32 slice computerized tomography (CT) and an MRI machine (**Fig. 4**).

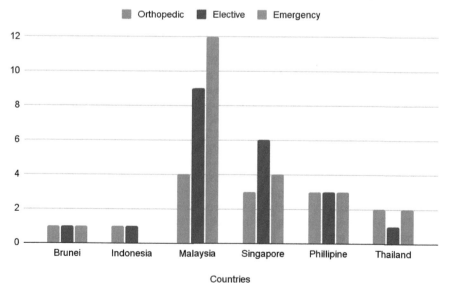

Fig. 3. Classification of various procedures conducted in exotic animal practices into 3 types (orthopedics, elective, and emergency) in SEA.

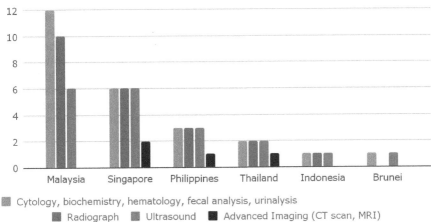

Fig. 4. Diagnostic capabilities of exotic animal practices in SEA.

DISCUSSION
Thailand

Historically, there has always been an abundance of wildlife and exotic pets kept as pets in Thailand but health care for these species have been lacking. Fifteen years ago, there were only 3 or 4 hospitals in Thailand that were able to see exotic pets. The increasing interest in exotic pets has been propelled by an aging society and urbanization.[6] Exotic pets have proved popular for decades due to easy accessibility and their appeal to customers with modern lifestyles. In 2022, the exotic pet market posted 16% growth, with small mammals constituting 64%, avian species 23%, reptiles 7%, and the remaining 6% attributed to other categories.[6] There are many social media platforms (www.pantip.com) where the public can share information about exotic pets, chat with the vet, and buy exotic pets from the Jatujak market (Bangkok's most extensive pet market). According to Euromonitor, the market value of pet care and pet food has consistently increased every year. In 2018, the pet business was valued at 31 billion baht.[6] The mindset of exotic pet owners has also changed compared to 20 years ago. Pets are now treated as family with owners having more accountability for providing good medical care.

Today, the landscape has changed, and many general hospitals can accept exotic pets. There are 5 to 10 exotics-focused mixed practices (with caseloads of 60%–70% exotic pets and 20%–30% dogs and cats) and 1 hospital that specializes in exotic pets only. The development of exotic pet medicine in Thailand is largely due to the contributions of the founders of the Zoo and Wildlife Association of Thailand, which was created 22 years ago. There are around 20 pioneer members, including zoologic instructors from the university and zoo vets. The association runs an annual 10 day zoo/wildlife training course for selected undergraduates from various universities. After 10 years, this has produced several veterinarians who ended up working as wildlife vets and exotic pet veterinarians. Some of these individuals also ended up in exotic teaching positions in universities (Appendix 3). The Thailand Exotic Pet Veterinarian Association (TEPVA) was then founded in 2015 by 2 members of the original association who have dedicated their careers as exotic pet veterinarians. This association has subsequently lobbied for the inclusion of exotic pet medicine and surgery at universities. They also organize exotic seminars and workshops by local and international speakers.

In the future, it is predicted that more vets will specialize in exotics to match the increasing demands. Referral hospitals with exotics departments are being established to accommodate this demand. There will be more subspecialization of vets with areas of interest such as veterinary acupuncture, ophthalmology, orthopedics, and urology. The Thai Vet Board already has its own College of Veterinary Specialties Veterinary Council of Thailand (VCT) with specialist diplomas in 5 major areas. There are plans to create an exotic pet medicine specialist diploma soon. Candidates for exotic pet medicine must pass a small animal internal medicine and subsequently an exotic medicine examination.

Philippines

The fascination with wildlife and zoo animals in the Philippines started when Manila Zoo opened its doors on July 25, 1959. This spurred interest in keeping exotic animals as pets. Private collectors would seek medical help initially from the veterinarians at Manila Zoo. In 1970, the Philippines Parks and Wildlife Center opened in Quezon City, and this was subsequently renamed as the National Wildlife Rescue and Research Center in 2011. This became the primary wildlife rescue center and also a mini-zoo. The rescue center also served as an establishment where people could get medical advice for their exotic pets. The demand in veterinary health care for exotic pets created interest for vet practitioners.

A Social Weather Stations survey of 1200 shows that 64% of Filipino households have pets at home, and it is not unusual to see more than one species in their households.[7] Filipinos have a natural interest in cats, dogs, birds, small mammals, and reptiles, and many treat them like their family members. The new generation of pet owners is generally more aware of the medical attention, welfare, and needs of their domestic and exotic pets. Pet owners are finding ways to improve their enclosures, nutrition, enrichments, and medical needs.

Over the years, the demand for exotic animal health, exotic pet food, and supply keeps increasing. The number of exotic clienteles has increased tremendously over the past 4 years, especially for small mammals and reptiles. With an increasing number of exotic pet shows/exhibits being organized for the public each year, more people are exposed to and are interested in exotic pet ownership. The challenges faced in the Philippines are similar in that many Filipino veterinarians are interested in exotic practice but unfortunately, there is limited access to certified training and education to pursue the specialization. With increasing demand in the practice, current exotic practitioners are starting to be overwhelmed. Moreover, pet owners with exotic pets from far away provinces have a difficult time seeking medical advice from exotic practitioners who are only located in Metro Manila.

The University of the Philippines College of Veterinary Medicine does offer some exotic/wildlife medicine training as part of the undergraduate curriculum. However, it was more theoretical due to limited access and distance to wildlife centers, zoos, and aquariums. Those with exotic animal interests can learn clinical skills and knowledge such as species identification, nutrition, and enclosure design from the National Wildlife Rescue and Research Center. They may also choose to do a rotation in Ocean Adventure, an aquarium with marine mammals. During the externship program in the last year of the undergraduate program, students can also elect to spend time working in other wildlife centers or exotic hospitals overseas to gain clinical experience. National associations for vets such as the Philippine Animal Hospital Association (PAHA) and Veterinary Practitioners Association of the Philippines

(VPAP) have also recently included wildlife and exotic medicine streams in their yearly conventions (Appendix 3).

There have been many advancements in the level of care of exotic practices in the Philippines over the last few years. However, there is still ongoing difficulty in obtaining exotic equipment locally, and there is limited access to pain medications and anesthetic drugs for both small animals and exotic/wildlife species. Most of the specific equipment for exotics must be imported from overseas. Exotic practitioners frequently improvise with different techniques to overcome these challenges. Diagnostics testing capabilities are improving but currently, there is no access to polymerase chain reaction testing for viral infections in reptiles, birds, and small mammals in the country.

Malaysia

Historically, exotic animal patients were not commonly presented in the clinic. In the early 1980s and 1990s, exotic animals such as rabbits, guinea pigs, and macaques were kept in research facilities, and they had no access to laboratory veterinarians. Veterinarians interested in exotics would be called upon for treatment, postmortems, and sample collections for research purposes. Until the early 2000s, law enforcement for wildlife and exotic animals was lacking. Local wildlife was regularly kept as pets. Livestock such as domestic chickens, geese, and ducks were also occasionally kept as pets. Other common exotic pets include rabbits, guinea pigs, and red-eared sliders. Many of the cases presented to veterinary clinics were related to inappropriate diet and husbandry due to a lack of client knowledge about the care of the animals due to the inaccessibility of information.

In the past, Malaysian vets faced many challenges when dealing with exotic pets. In the 1980s and 1990s, exotic animals were often treated with limited diagnostic tests due to financial constraints and the unwillingness of the client to spend on animals that are perceived of low value. Another major factor is the limited training that veterinarians receive for exotic medicine including lack of training to collect diagnostic samples from exotic species. In some cases, radiographs were carried out for patients, but interpretation was challenging. There was no expertise to interpret hematology slides, and no machines were available to be calibrated for values other than for domestic cats, dogs, ruminants, and horses. The majority of exotic cases were only offered outpatient treatments, and surgeries were seldom performed. Limited veterinary drugs are available for use as its legislation comes under the pharmacy department, which is a subsidiary of the Ministry of Health. The lack of understanding of the need for the utilization of certain veterinary drugs has resulted in the prohibition of common veterinary drugs including anesthetics and vaccines.

There have been many upheavals over the last 15 years. There is improved economic stability and increased client spending and interest in keeping exotic pets. Social media has also captivated the public creating a big interest in keeping exotic animals in Malaysia. There are fluctuations in the trends in keeping certain species depending on the popularity among influencers. Training opportunities for veterinarians have become available in the 2 universities with veterinary medicine programs (Universiti Putra Malaysia in Serdang, Selangor and Universiti Kelantan Malaysia, Kelantan) since the establishment of a wildlife and exotic unit in the teaching hospitals. Since the last decade, exotic animal medicine courses have become compulsory curriculums for the veterinary medicine program. The establishment of the Association for Wildlife and Exotic Medicine and Wildlife and Exotic Veterinarian Special Interest Group (WEVSIG) in 2021 has helped improve exotic animal practice in Malaysia (Appendix 3). WEVSIG was established by practicing veterinarians from zoos, clinicians from private clinics, wildlife rescue centers, and aquariums. In the last 2 years,

WEVSIG produced newsletters and organized webinars, conferences, and workshops for exotic and wildlife medicine. There have been high numbers of participation from exotic practitioners in private practices indicating a great interest in this field. The WEVSIG task force assembles subject experts of exotic/wildlife veterinarians in the country to assist in complex cases when needed. There are currently no specialist certifications or residency programs for exotic medicine. Veterinarians wishing to study further about exotic medicine can pursue a postgraduate program in the 2 veterinary schools in Malaysia. These research-based graduate programs have limited clinical components with occasional involvement in handling exotics during the collection of samples for their dissertations. Researchers would focus on studies such as disease surveillance among wildlife[8] or pharmacologic studies in exotic species.[9]

The future of exotic animal veterinarians in Malaysia appears promising. With the advancement of information technology in the last 25 years, exotic practitioners can easily keep abreast with the latest knowledge through online forums, exotic pet care sites, and online veterinary courses. In addition to local universities providing ongoing continuing education training programs, there are also exotic medicine streams in regional small animal associations conferences such as the Malaysian Small Animal Veterinarian Association, Federation of Small Animal Association, and World Small Animal Associations. We hope that the proposed shift for the veterinary drugs laws from the current jurisdiction to the Department of Veterinary Services under the Ministry of Agriculture will lead to the approval of important and relevant veterinary drugs. Increased cooperation between the authorities, universities, veterinary associations, and clinicians will also heighten awareness of illegal wildlife trading thus improving exotic animal welfare.

Singapore

Singapore has a unique situation as a small and modern city, with a fairly recent history of veterinary industry development. There is no veterinary school in Singapore. The first veterinary scholars were sent abroad to study by the government in the 1950s with the sole purpose of returning to work for the government to care for livestock in the public health sector. Many worked at the pig and poultry research institute and the central veterinary laboratory to develop management and disease control in pig farming. Pig farming was phased out in 1990 due to land constraints and pollution. In the 1970s, there was only 1 government-run small animal veterinary clinic in the country until the first privately owned clinic opened in 1975. In 1978, there were a total of 3 clinics that treated mainly dogs and cats with minimal focus on exotic pets.[10] In the 1960s to 1970s before Singapore became a signatory of the Convention of International Trade in Endangered Species of Wild Fauna and Flora (CITES), it was not uncommon to find private collections of a variety of exotic animals, even orangutans and other non-human primates, civet cats, and a variety of large feline species. In the 1970s to 1980s, these pets declined as the numbers of large private land parcels were requisitioned by the government and regulations made it illegal to keep them. The implementation of the CITES and the Wildlife Act[11] and Endangered Species (Import and Export) Act[12] from 1965 to 1989 greatly impacted exotic animal ownership. There is now a very short list of exotic species that can be kept as pets in Singapore. The only exotic companion animals allowed are rabbits, mice, hamsters, gerbils, guinea pigs, and chinchillas. Reptiles and amphibians permitted are limited to the red-eared sliders, Malayan box turtles, green tree frogs, American bullfrogs, crab-eating frogs, and land hermit crabs. The restrictions on avian species appear less stringent with the only illegal species including hornbills, eagles, falcons, vultures, hawks, blue-crowned hanging parrot, blue-rumped parrot, straw-headed bulbul, and any local native or feral wildlife species.[11] Some owners still smuggle or buy illegal exotic animals from underground traders, but the numbers are unknown.

In the last 2 decades, the number of legal exotic pet owners has grown dramatically. Ninety percent of Singaporean residents live in small apartments, which makes the keeping of large and noisy species more challenging. Small exotic mammals and small birds gained popularity due to their nature allowing them to be confined in small areas. The 1990s saw a spike in ownership of rabbits, chinchillas, and hamsters. From 2014 to 2019, exotic small mammal ownership increased from 85,900 to 92,300.[13] This trend was largely due to influences from social media and the formation of exotic interest groups such as House Rabbit Society Singapore, Guinea Pig Rescue Singapore, Hamster Society Singapore, and Little Hammy Rescue Singapore. These volunteer-run groups actively help increase public awareness of basic husbandry, diets, and common diseases of rabbits, guinea pigs, and hamsters. They also advocate for good health care and veterinary wellness examinations. The groups actively rescue sick animals and encourage veterinarians to see exotics. Over the years, they have influenced the public to present exotic animals to preferred exotic vets hence growing the demand for exotic veterinary health services. With the advent of the Internet, there is also improved access to formulated diets for exotics, specialized housing, and equipment as well as husbandry information. Freshwater fish such as arowana, flowerhorn cichlids, and red-eared have also gained popularity among owners due to their accessibility and prominence in local cultural beliefs. Due to a tropical climate all year round, koi ponds are also popular among wealthy owners, but koi fish are mostly seen as ornamental water features. Health care for fish is still a developing field with many fish hobbyists consulting aquarists for treatment and even surgeries.

Veterinary health care for exotics in Singapore was initially lacking even in the early 2000s. Many vets struggled with the skills and knowledge to treat these species due to limited resources and training available. Traditionally, there has not been much financial motivation to see exotics. Many veterinarians charged less for exotic pet services so that they were able to learn from the cases and help care for the pets. Illegal exotic pets are seldom presented to the veterinarian due to the owners' fear of getting reported and subsequent confiscation of illegal pets. Many veterinarians are reluctant to get involved due to laws that would penalize the vets for not reporting illegal species. Most illnesses tend to be due to diet and husbandry issues likely because of the lack of information about their care.

Singapore is now considered a first-world country. It is highly developed with a successful economy, advanced infrastructure, and a high standard of living for its residents. It is an extremely expensive city to live in. Many exotic pet owners have excellent spending power, and pets are treated very well. Most owners are willing to spend on medical expenses when necessary. The latest survey in 2022 shows that there are 100 private veterinary practices and 450 licensed veterinarians in the public and private sectors in the country. Out of these, around 8 to 10 practices will see exotic animals. Three emergency hospitals will see exotics for any overnight emergencies. In the last 10 years, more veterinarians can diagnose and treat exotic pets as many clinics and hospitals are well equipped with diagnostic equipment such as in-house blood tests, radiography, and ultrasonography. Many veterinarians have access to exotics textbooks, online continuing education, and forums such as the Veterinary Information Network. The referral exotics practice established 4 years ago provides the opportunity for exotic pet practitioners to refer and transfer cases to an ABVP exotics companion mammal specialist. The level of veterinary care for exotics has seen a great improvement and intensive care hospitalization for exotic animals is commonly offered. With access to an array of diagnostic services such as computed tomography, MRI, cardiology, and ultrasound services, the ability to treat and diagnose diseases in exotic animals has exponentially improved. Advanced soft tissue surgeries and orthopedic repairs are commonly performed on exotic pets by the exotic companion medicine (ECM) specialist and a board-certified surgeon. Continuing education lectures for exotics have been taught by the ECM specialist at the local Singapore Veterinary Association conferences, veterinary nursing school as well as the hospital's own continuing education (CE) talks, organized for Singaporean veterinarians. International conferences such as the Singapore Vet Show and the World Small Animal Veterinary Association (WSAVA) conferences held in Singapore have an exotic stream with talks by invited international exotics specialists.

The landscape for exotic animal practice in Singapore still faces some challenges. The dissemination of exotic veterinary knowledge is still lacking for veterinarians, and information available to the public is often misleading. This is, in part, due to the lack of a veterinary association focusing on exotic pets. Legislation to control the type of exotic pets does limit the exposure of exotic practitioners to treat a wide range of exotic animal species. Many illegal species may suffer poor health care due to the reluctance of the owner to engage in veterinary services. This law does create frustrations for exotic veterinarians and inevitably results in difficulty in attracting more exotic specialists to work in Singapore. Over-the-counter drugs are still available in pet shops and aquariums for many exotic pets such as fish and birds. This results in a lot of self-treatment by owners instead of engaging veterinary professionals. Many exotic pet clients in Singapore are very active in the exotic animal interest groups and forums that have the advantage of fostering a strong community of animal lovers. However, since discussions are led by pet owners, recommendations for veterinary care, husbandry, and diet may often be biased and inaccurate.

Improving the future of veterinary services for exotic pets will rely on several factors. The formation of a veterinary association focusing on exotic veterinary medicine appears prudent to lead the dissemination of information on exotic pet care and provide continuing education for the veterinary community. Also, collaboration with government bodies should be considered given certain legislation on exotic animal practices. There should be a tightening of control of oxytetracycline (OTC) drugs available for fish and birds and a law preventing aquarists in pet shops and fish farms from treating fish without a veterinarian's supervision. There should be leniencies in the type of exotic pets allowed for ownership based on what is ethically acceptable and also based on conservation laws. The recent establishment of an American Board of Veterinary Practitioners (ABVP) ECM residency program in Singapore in 2023 is a promising change as it will help grow the pool of specialized exotic vets.

Indonesia

The owners of exotic pets in Indonesia were historically more inclined to self-treat exotic pets rather than seek professional veterinary assistance. This was, in part, due to a lack of veterinarians who were confident in treating exotics and could not even perform examinations on exotic animals. However, presently, in Indonesia today, many owners are starting to keep exotic animals not just as pets but as family members. Many would visit veterinarians for examinations for wellness checkups and seek veterinary treatment when pets fall ill. The development of exotic medicine in Indonesia is currently growing rapidly. Exotic animal owners are starting to understand and pay attention to the importance of routine examinations and preventive health care. Currently, there are many more exotic pet practitioners, many of which have good reputations and improved accessibility to a good standard of pet health care.

The Veterinary Medical Association for Wildlife, Aquatic, and Exotic Animals (ASLI-QEWAN) was established in 2000 and helped spearhead the education of Indonesian vets on the health management of wildlife and exotic animals. Seminars were first held from July to August 2000 and have continued since then. The Veterinary Communication Forum for wildlife and exotic animal veterinarians was founded shortly after this to organize continuing education for veterinarians to improve their knowledge and skills for wildlife and exotic animals. In 2003, training in exotic medicine was introduced through seminars and workshops. The response of veterinarians in Indonesia was quite positive to learn this new field of science. The Faculty of Veterinary Medicine in Indonesian universities also began to introduce modules on exotic animal and wildlife health management for the undergraduate course. In recent years, the number of exotic animal practitioners in Indonesia has grown very rapidly. The demand for seminars, webinars, and workshops with the theme of exotic animal medicine is always in high demand. Fortunately, the distribution of exotic animal practitioners is increasingly evenly distributed throughout Indonesia to match the demand for health care for exotic species in this large populous country.

SUMMARY

Despite challenges faced by exotic practitioners in many SEA countries, the trend over the last few decades appears to be promising with the standard of veterinary care for exotics improving. Due to the advancement of information technology, many vets can now access continuing education online. There are also many regional exotics training courses and better access to leaders in the field for referrals and discussion of cases. Further collaboration among exotic vets through veterinary interest organizations for exotic animals in SEA will help with the dissemination of knowledge and improve the level of knowledge of exotic animal practice in SEA.

CLINICS CARE POINTS

- In many SEA countries, the development of exotic animal health care stemmed from knowledge and training provided by local zoo and wildlife veterinarians.
- This has translated to future generations of competent exotic pet veterinarians with many pioneering the path of future exotic pet practitioners.
- Traditionally, the only way to achieve board specialization has been through internationally recognized board certifications for exotic pets in the United Kingdom, Australia, or the United States. This is challenging for many individuals to relocate overseas to get training abroad and the language barrier may also add a level of complexity.
- There has been some progress in establishing recognized structured certifications in exotic animal pet practice in some SEA countries.
- There are many more accessible learning opportunities available for exotic pet practitioners with the advent of online continuing education, which has helped bridge the gap in knowledge in exotic pet practice.

ACKNOWLEDGMENTS

The authors would like to thank the following exotic practitioners for providing valuable information about the exotic animal practice in their countries: Dr Chaowaphan Yinharnmingmongkol, Dr Cathy Chan, Dr Frederic Chua, Dr Hsu Li Chieh, Dr Wendy Chee, Associate prof Dr Vellayan Subramaniam, Dr Abraham Gabriel, Dr Brenda

Gilbert, Dr Napoleon Manuel Almelor, Dr Muhammad Ridwan, Dr Muhammad Reza Ramadhani, Dr Jaffar Abdul Jabar, and Dr Slamet Rahardjo.

DISCLOSURE

The authors have nothing to disclose.

REFERENCES

1. Hughes AC. Mapping priorities for conservation in Southeast Asia. Biol Conserv 2017;209:395–405.
2. Bush ER, Baker SE, Macdonald DW. Global trade in exotic pets 2006–2012. Conserv Biol 2014;28(3):663–76.
3. Hill H. The political economy of policy reform: insights from Southeast Asia. In: Coxhead I, editor. Routledge Handbook of Southeast Asian economics. New York, NY: Routledge; 2014. p. 327–44.
4. Timo K. The long peace of ASEAN. J Peace Res 2001;38(1):5–25.
5. Nijman V, Morcatty T, Smith JH, et al. Illegal wildlife trade–surveying open animal markets and online platforms to understand the poaching of wild cats. Biodivers 2019;20(1):58–61.
6. Jitpleecheep P. Duo team up for exotic pet hospital. Bangkok Post. 2023. Available at: https://www.bangkokpost.com/business/general/2705748/duo-team-up-for-exotic-pet-hospital. [Accessed 28 December 2023].
7. Marcelino A. SWS: Pets In 64% Filipino households, plants in 67%. Inquirer.net. Published September 29, 2023. Available at: https://newsinfo.inquirer.net/1838643/survey-says-64-of-filipino-households-have-pets-67-have-plants. Accessed December 28, 2023.
8. Gilbert B. Molecular identification and Zoonotic Potential of SARS-CoV-2-like Viruses in Bats from East Coast, Peninsular Malaysia, Dissertation. Kelantan, Malaysia: Universiti Malaysia Kelantan; 2023.
9. Gabriel A. Clinical Evaluation of Antibiotic Loaded Calcium Phosphate (Alcap) Beads as prophylaxis and treatment options for avian soft tissue and orthopedic cases. Dissertation. Universiti Putra Malaysia; 2018.
10. Ngiam TT, Chua T, Lim K, et al. Vets at work: Tracing the progress of veterinarians in Singapore. Singapore: Singapore Veterinary Association; 2022.
11. Wildlife Act 1965 revised 2000 revision (Singapore) ch 351 s 5C. Available at: https://www.nparks.gov.sg/-/media/avs/legislations/wildlife-act-(chapter-351).pdf?la=en&hash=491A76EE1BB64BEA4EC7BD9A85F70A2067B9F209. [Accessed 28 November 2023].
12. Endangered Species (Import and Export) Act revised 2008 (Singapore) ch 92A,s 4. Available at: https://www.nparks.gov.sg/-/media/avs/legislations/(3a)-endangered-species-(import-and-export)-act.ashx. [Accessed 28 November 2023].
13. Lam F, Tay V. Paws-perous business: the booming pets trade that's also feeding an illicit market. The Business Times. Published January 11, 2020. Available at: https://www.businesstimes.com.sg/opinion-features/features/paws-perous-business-booming-pets-trade-thats-also-feeding-illicit-market. [Accessed 20 December 2023].

Appendix 1

APPENDIX 1: LIST OF SELECTED DIAGNOSTIC LABORATORIES FOR EXOTIC PETS IN SOUTHEAST ASIA

Selected Diagnostic Laboratories for Exotic Pets	
Country	Name of Laboratory
Malaysia	*Innoquest Pathology Sdn. Bhd* Headquarters Office 2nd Floor, Wisma Tecna 18A, Jalan 51 A/223 46100 Petaling Jaya Phone (International): +603 7841 7752 Web site: https://www.innoquest.com.my/ *Universiti Putra Malaysia* Veterinary Laboratory Services 43,400 UPM Serdang Selangor Darul Ehsan Web site: https://vet.upm.edu.my/department/veterinary_pathology_ microbiology/laboratory_services-1164 *PATHLAB Laboratory Malaysia* Pathlab Headquarter Wisma KAM, 97–91, Jalan SS25/2, Taman Bukit Emas 47,301 Petaling Jaya, Selangor Darul Ehsan, Malaysia Phone: +603 7882 26888 Web site: https://www.pathlab.com.my/
Singapore	*ANTECH/Asia Veterinary Diagnostics* 83 Genting Lane, #05–02A Genting Building Singapore 349568 Phone: +65 6291 5412 Email: sg@avd.asia Web site: https://avd.asia/ *BioAcumen Global Pte Ltd* 158 Kallang Way, #05–08/09/10, Singapore 349245 Phone: +65 6592 2336 Email: sales@bioacumen.com Web site: https://bioacumen.com/ *IDEXX Laboratories Singapore* 21 Biopolis Road Nucleos (North Tower) #03–06, Singapore 138567 Phone: +65 6807 6288 Fax: +65 6397 5279 Web site: https://www.idexx.com/en/
Philippines	*Vet Central Lab* Ground Floor, Units B&C, One Roxas Squaire #1F. Roxas cor R. Blumentritt, Brgy Tibagan San Juan City, Manila, Philippines Phone: +63 2852 5081 Email: vetcentrallabphils@gmail.com *Advanced Diagnostic Veterinary Laboratories (DVL)* Phone number: (02) 850–1861 Mobile number: +639178835719 Email address: dvlabs@abclab.com.ph and dvl_sales@abclab.com.ph Address: LG-1 Richville Corporate Tower, Madrigal Business Park, Ayala-Alabang, Muntinlupa City, Philippines

(continued on next page)

(continued)

Selected Diagnostic Laboratories for Exotic Pets	
Country	**Name of Laboratory**
Thailand	*Vet Central Lab* 148,150 Tiwanon Road, Bang Kraso Subdistrict, Mueang District, Nonthaburi Province 11000. Tel. 081-4007929, 0-2591-8013-16 Fax 0-2591-8015-6 Web site: http://www.vetcentrallab.com/ *Vet and Vitro Central Lab (RAMKHAMHAENG)* 2/69 The Wayra (Ramkhamhaeng-Suwannabhumi) Ratpattana Road, Saphansung, Bangkok, 10240 Thailand Phone: +662-046-4991 Fax: +662-046-4991 ext 14 Web site: https://www.vetandvitro.co.th/th/ Email: Vetramkhamhaeng@vetandvitro.co.th *Vet Clinical Center* 324-326 Phlapphlachai Road, Pom Prap Subdistrict, Pom Prap Sattru Phai District, Bangkok, Thailand Phone: 095 571 1155 Email: vetclinicalcenter@gmail.com *Mahidol University* *Faculty of Veterinary Science: The Center for Veterinary Diagnosis* 999 Phutthamonthon Sai 4 Road, Salaya, Phutthamonthon, Nakhonpathom, 73170 Thailand Faculty of Veterinary Science: 02-441-5242 Email: vdc.vetmu@gmail.com
Indonesia	*IPB University* *School of Veterinary Medicine & Biomedical Sciences* *Education and Services Laboratory* Address: Jl. Agatis IPB Dramaga, Bogor Phone: (+62) 251 8471 431 Email: skhb@apps.ipb.ac.id Web site: https://svmbs.ipb.ac.id/education-and-services-laboratory-lpl/ *Center for Primate Animal Studies (Pusat Study Satwa Primata)* Address: Jalan Lodaya II No.5, Babakan, Central Bogor, Babakan, Central Bogor District, Bogor City, West Java 16151 Phone: (0251)8320417 Email: @apps.ipb.ac.id Web site: https://primata-ipb-ac-id

Appendix 2

APPENDIX 2: LIST OF VETERINARY ASSOCIATIONS SUPPORTING EXOTIC ANIMAL VETERINARIANS IN SOUTHEAST ASIA

List of Exotic Veterinary Associations in SEA	
Malaysia	Wildlife & Exotic Veterinarian Special Interest Group (WEVSIG) Web site: https://sites.google.com/view/wevsig Instagram: https://www.instagram.com/wevsig21/

(continued on next page)

(continued)	
Thailand	*Thailand Exotic Pet Veterinarian Association (TEPVA)* Address: No. 141/1 Phutthamonthon Sai 2 Rd. Sala Thammasop Subdistrict, Thawi Watthana District, Bangkok, 10170 Mobile phone: +66 97 165 1100 Email: atepvs2016@gmail.com *The Veterinary Practitioner Association of Thailand (VPAT)* Address: 559/2 Praditmanuthum Road, Saphan Song, Wang Thong Lang, Bangkok 10310 Email: vpatthailand@gmail.com Web site: https://www.vpatthailand.org/ce-vpat-exotic Facebook: https://www.facebook.com/groups/125230494185964
Philippines	*Philippines Animal Hospital Association (PAHA)* Web site: https://paha.com.ph/ Facebook: https://www.facebook.com/PhilippineAnimalHospitalAssociationInc/ *Veterinary Practitioners Association of the Philippines (VPAP)* Web site: https://vpap.com.ph/ Facebook: https://www.facebook.com/vpap1972/
Indonesia	*The Veterinary Medical Association for Wildlife, Aquatic, and Exotic Animals (ASLIQEWAN)* Email: asliqewan@gmail.com Instagram: https://www.instagram.com/asliqewan/?hl=en

Appendix 3

APPENDIX 3: LIST OF QUESTIONS IN ONLINE SURVEY QUESTIONNAIRE

Name of clinical practice   Southeast Asia (SEA) country that you are practicing as a veterinarian
Name of veterinary school that you graduated from, and which country is the school located in?   Number of years of undergraduate degree
Did your undergraduate program cover exotic animal practice/zoologic medicine as part of your veterinary training?
Yes/No   If applicable, can you list the details of exotics/zoologic medicine training you received in your undergraduate program?

Did you receive any formal postgraduate training (eg, internship and residency) for exotic animal practice/zoologic medicine?
    Do you regularly attend structured continuing education (CE) for exotics species?
    Yes/No

Can you give details of CE you attend (eg, Exoticscon, distance learning courses, local workshop)?   Do you do self-directed learning for exotics species? If yes, can you list the details?

Are you a member if any association/club for exotics medicine and surgery? If yes, can you list the name of association(s)/club(s)?
Do you have any formal specialist board certificates for any exotics species?
Yes/No

If applicable, can you list the specialist board certificates you obtained for exotics species
Which of the option below describes your current breakdown of clinical caseload?
Exotics only
Mainly exotics and some dogs/cats
Mainly dogs/cats and some exotics

Which exotics species do you see in your clinical practice? You can choose more than 1 option below:

Birds

Reptiles

Amphibians

Exotics small mammals (eg, Rabbits, guinea pigs, hamsters, chinchillas, degus, mice, rats, sugar gliders, and hedgehogs)

Large cats

Primates

Fish

Others (not listed)
Do you see venomous snakes in your practice?
Yes/No

What is the percentage breakdown of the presenting complaint for veterinary visit? Please specify the percentage the cases seen in this order below:

General Health Checks

Illness

Emergency

Others (please elaborate)
Is overnight hospitalization available for exotic animals at your practice?
Yes/No

Which of the following hospital facilities are available for exotics animals? You can choose more than 1 option below:

Heat cages/incubators

Oxygen chamber

Electrocardiogram monitoring machine

Pulse oximetry

Fluid pumps for intravenous (IV) fluids

Gavage/crop needles for birds

Snake handling equipment
Do you provide emergency consults for exotics species during your operational hours?
Yes/No

If yes, are you able to provide 24 hours emergency consults?

Yes/No
What are your alternative options for clients if 24 hours emergency service/walk in is not available at your practice/facility?

What are the diagnostics modalities/equipment do you commonly used for exotics animals? You can choose more than 1 option below:

Radiography

Ultrasound

Computerized tomography (CT)

MRI

In-house blood biochemistry panel

In-house complete blood count (CBC)

Rigid endoscopy

Laparoscopy

Cytology

Parasitology
   Do you engage a radiology service for imaging interpretation for example, radiograph/CT scan? If yes, can you provide the name of the company?

Do you perform microbiology? If yes, which external laboratory service do you send your samples to?
   Do you perform elective surgery/procedure for exotics in your clinical practice? If yes, can you elaborate more? (eg, castration, spay for rabbits)

Do you perform orthopedic surgeries in your practice?

Yes/No

Exotic Animal Practice in South Asia

Shiwani D. Tandel, BVSc & AH, MVSc, MVetSci (Cons med)

KEYWORDS

- South asia • Indian subcontinent • Vedas • Shailhotra • Elephants

KEY POINTS

- This manuscript is a narrative of the evolution of exotic animal medicine in South Asia, though the ages.
- Traditionally ayurvedic medicine evolved in India and this science was and continues to be used to treat animals as an adjunct to allopathic medicnes.
- There is an effort to try to weave traditional folklore and beliefs into the current environment of the trend of keeping exotic pets.
- It also examines how veterinary schools and provate practitioners are adapting tothe growing popularity of exotic pets, showcasing efforts to enhance education and practice for this novel stream of veterinary medicine.

Veterinary medicine in South Asia has been recorded 4000 years ago, where the sages have recorded in the Vedas, methods to treat domestic and animals used in warfare like elephants and carrier pigeons. Understanding the history of evolution of veterinary medicine in India is equally important when we speak about exotic animal practice. Veterinary medicine was practiced by Salutri's, a name synonymous with a veterinarian in the post Vedic times.[1]

IRON AGE 1100 BC TO 300 BC

The early sages used the age old traditional Ayurveda to treat animals. According to Hindu scriptures, Charak and Sushrut Samhita, discuss animal disease and their treatments. Ayurveda is primarily plant derived medicine, which originated by its students after studying 'higher beings'(animals) consuming plants or root. They believe these animals were guided by their intrinsic knowledge to heal the body. This information was recorded in books like the Atharva Samhita.[2] There are chapters dedicated to veterinary medicine and remedies used for certain ailments. This maybe restricted to domestic animals but there is a mention of species of fowl and elephants, whose diseases and treatments were also included.[3] Priests or Rishi's were the first

Phoenix Veterinary Specialty, 2,3 Vipin Residency, Gokhale Road, Dadar, Mumbai 400028, India
E-mail address: shiwani.tandel@gmail.com

Vet Clin Exot Anim 27 (2024) 551–560
https://doi.org/10.1016/j.cvex.2024.03.008
1094-9194/24/© 2024 Elsevier Inc. All rights reserved.

veterinarians of ancient India. Prominent among those were Shalihotra—earliest expert in horse medicine and author of 'Haya Ayurveda'— and Palakapya,author of Hasty–Ayurveda-elephant medicine. These 2 species were very closely worked on along with cows because horses and elephants were used as war animals. This treaty prescribed medicines for jaundice, constipation of the bowel, fainting/swooning, headache, dysentery, paralysis, inflammation, skin disease, colic pain, and intestinal tumor of domesticated elephants. It also suggests ideal meals for them during normal/war/famine times.[2,4] These were some of the earliest reports of wild/exotic animal medicine practice in the country.

Historical Age – After 300 BC

Veterinary doctors during the Mauryan empire videlicet during 300 BC[5] were aware of the science of domestic and non-domestic species. There were many texts written, which explains animal keeping and ayurvedic medicine with different techniques. The text 'Krishi-Parashar', which literally means agriculture by Saint Parashar, deals with domestic animal medicine, it emphasizes about correct housing practices with dimensions for cattle, horses, and elephants,[6] The text Agni- Purana describes fumigation of cow houses with vapors of Viosha, Devdaru (Deodar tree), hing (asophodita), mustard seed, and guggul (bdellium tree) mixture to prevent spread of contagious disease. The text Arthashastra, described the size, orientation, and sanitization system of the royal horse and elephant sheds.[7] These medical treatments suggested by ancient Indian literacy can be very useful for animal keepers in remote rural parts of the country, where veterinary help cannot reach.[8]

Islamic Rule and The Medieval Period – 1100 to 1850 AD

An Italian traveler, Pietro dela Valle-sailed from Venice to India in the early 17th century and described a bird hospital in Cambay, present day Khambat in Gujarat. This was a hospital dedicated only to birds as early as 1539, the 16th century. Injured migratory birds were bought in here. The excerpt says, 'The house of this hospital is small, a little room sufficing for many birds: yet I saw it full of birds of all sorts, which needed attendance, as cocks, hens, pigeons, peacocks, ducks, and small birds, which during their being lame or sick, or mateless are kept there, but being recovered and in good plight, if they be wild they are let go at liberty; if domestic they are given to some pious person who keeps them in his house (sic). This place was maintained on public alms.'[9]

British Colonisation – 18th and 19th Century

But it was during the British rule when animals were actually collected for entertainment purposes or to be added to personal collections. These collections were then called zoos. They were predominantly collections owned by princely states or authorities from the British army who were in a commanding position to be able to keep such collections. The first zoo was established in Barrackpore in 1801, built by Lord Wellesley in the 19th century. The zoo had animals such as the African donkey, tiger, bear, bison, leopard, mouse deer, kangaroos, monkeys, and various species of birds.[10] Lord Wellesley felt the need of making a detailed description of the animals in Asia. This was primarily because the Europeans were mostly ignorant when it came to the category of Indian animals. He started working on the first Natural Research Center in Asia, the 'National Heritage of India'. Various animals were required to be collected. Barrackpore Zoo was built to store these animals and birds. Until 1804, 2791 was invested in the cost of maintenance of these animals and birds.[10]

The animals suffering from illness at the zoos were treated by veterinarians who were treating the animals in the army. The first veterinary training school was established in Pune for the mounted corps.[11] Traditionally, animals in zoos were earlier kept for entertainment purposes and veterinarians were sourced if the need arose. But eventually as the need increased, formal veterinary education in India began in 1862, with the establishment of army veterinary school in Pune. Fifteen years after that the first civil veterinary school was started in Babugarh (Harpur), in UP in 1877 and a college was started in Lahore in 1882. The curriculum supported treating animals required for agriculture. When production animals started suffering from epidemics, there was need for a veterinary laboratory. Indian Veterinary Research Institute was established in 1889 in Pune and then it was moved to Mukhteshwar. This move was so that scientists could work safely with pathogenic viruses like Rinderpest away from crowded places. Veterinary colleges were associated with agricultural universities and were established with the sole intent to support the agriculture industry.

EMERGENCE OF WILD ANIMAL MEDICINE

Exotic animal medicine is very closely related to the growth of wildlife medicine in India. India is a biodiverse region and there is a flagship species in every biota. Historically, when the Portuguese and British came to India, there are reports of offering animals as gifts by the traders to the Indian princely states to continue trade in the region. There are reports of Malawi (African) traders bringing a giraffe to Bengal to present it as a gift to royalty there. Exotic animals and birds were thus introduced through trade during those times. There is no historical information about how these animals were cared for but since the knowledge of Ayurveda was prevalent during those times, it is presumed that in case of illness they were looked after by the 'vaid' or court physician.

In 1952, post-independence the Indian Board for wildlife was set up.[12] Prior to this, there were a few state level boards that were set up to protect wild animals in the region. The board had a strong mandate for zoos and created a zoo wing and a bird wing to conduct regular meetings. Soon the need for an association was felt to discuss problems in zoo administration, find methods for improvement of existing zoos, and to assess the scientific, educational, recreational aesthetic value of zoos in the community life of the nation. This led to the formation of an All India Zoo Association. Finally, in 1973, the zoo wing was replaced by the Expert committee, which was the precursor to the Zoo Authority or current Central Zoo authority. The Indian Wildlife Protection Act was passed in 1972, which stated that no Indian fauna can be kept in captivity by a private collector unless they have permission by law. They segregated Indian species into Schedules 1 to 4 in accordance with their population numbers and importance in conservation. This act made provisions for zoos and museums, with special reference to capture and trophies.[12] It also addressed the different formats under which animals were held in captive situations. Especially, since some zoos were outgrowths of animal holding facilities constructed to keep the animals rescued or trapped for different reasons or confiscated from people holding them illegally. There were 'traveling zoos', which might have been in existence for a long time, as it was a family business most of the times of the people who participated in animal trapping.[12] Some zoos were founded to hold royal collections. Some specialist collections such as snake parks were found by individuals interested in reptiles.[12] In 1988, a zoo consultancy project was initiated by the Wildlife Institute of India and in continuation a training course for Zoo Personnel.[12] This was the time when wildlife veterinarians got their own specialization. The mandate for the program was for in situ breeding and care of animals, but a small portion of this training was decided to health of wild animals kept in zoos, some of which were exotic species too. This was a turning point in wildlife medicine whereexotic animal medicine was slowly creeping into the foray as a specialty. Since establishing contact across the country was not as simple as it today, there were concentrated efforts by veterinarians located in geographically similar areas to concur on their wildlife problems. For example, in Assam there were veterinarians who specialized at treating rhinos; in Kerala- elephants; in Madhya Pradesh- tigers; and that is where veterinarians started getting 'species specialization' by experience. But, the experience has been limited to a particular set of maladies, for example, trauma, wounds, and seasonal diseases. No one really knows everything, as most of the experience came on the job. So every zoo and wildlife sanctuary had species specialist depending on their location but there weren't any efforts taken to find solutions to problems for all the animals since their numbers and species varied from zoo to zoo. Plus the number of veterinarians to animals was severely skewed. Therefore, some zoos did very well with some species and ignored the ailments of the ones they did not have confidence with. Sadly, because birds were too fragile, not many people could handle them and they have been the most neglected species; second-only to reptiles who have been the most ignored because they did well mostly, till they did not and then it was too late!

INCEPTION OF EXOTIC ANIMAL MEDICINE INTO THE SUBCONTINENT

Dr. Shiwani Tandel, the author of this article, finished her B.V.Sc & A.H from the Bombay Veterinary college in 2004 and that was a time when there was absolutely no one doing Avian and exotic animal medicine in the country. Veterinary Colleges were still under the agricultural university. When looking for conferences on wildlife medicine, the author came across the Association of Avian Veterinarians (AAV) conference website. This was in the year 2005, and the conference was supposed to be held at Monterey Bay, California. After returning from the conference and she spoke to my colleagues about the possibility of diagnosis and treatment for parrots. They didn't believe that there would be a market for such a specialty in India. Routinely, Indian Ringnecks, Hill mynahs, and Alexandrine parakeets were kept in Indian households as single birds for their speaking ability. It was a notion that the best talking parrot was generally a bird, which devoured green chillies. It was a routine practice to feed a primary diet of guava and chillies to the parrots. Not many people were informed about the legal aspects of keeping such birds and no one really cared. Although laws were in place, the commonly found fauna, which were in schedule 4 of the Wildlife Protection Act, were not considered noteworthy. Before the Wildlife Act was ammended in 2022, all the Indian wildlife were listed into 4 schedules, depending upon their status by the Convention on International Trade in Endangered Species of Wild Flora and Fauna. However, in 2022 all Indian wildlife was listed only in schedule 1 and schedule 2, both of which do not allow capturing, keeping, or hunting native wildlife.[13] However, ringnecks and alexandrine parakeets being extremely hardy never faced the need to go to a veterinarian. Since there were no vaccines for birds or reptiles for that matter, and diseases were identified too late or not at all. After consulting and gaining experience, the author turned to private practice. During those times being an only veterinary at the practice was acceptable and possible. In 2009, her clinic was the only clinic in India with a primary focus on exotic animal. They used to get very few birds as patients because of the lack of awareness of treatment possibilities. The breakthrough came for her when distributor of dog food realized that there was a need for packaged bird food in the Indian market. There were some bird fanciers who had very large collections of up to 2000 or 3000 birds. Distributors saw these as untapped markets and in order to introduce the food to breeders and collectors, they introduced the author as a veterinarian with an interest in avian and exotics. Not everyone accepted the idea of someone as young would be competent enough, to treat birds. They did not feel the need of a veterinarian or rather they did not know what they were missing and whether it was possible to treat this species, which they considered fragile. However, there were some breeders who allowed the author to visit them. At first hesitantly and then readily, when they saw the benefit, she got a golden opportunity to visit different aviaries across the country and gained hands on experience on the job. She had access to literature but had no mentor and she considered AAV her university. Going to conferences was expensive, but she sought help from her father who funded her trips to the Unites States. She gained a lot of knowledge from interacting with delegates at conferences. Veterinarians abroad were kind to offer short observer-ships and she was lucky to secure a chance to intern at the falcon hospital in Dubai. It was an exciting phase in her life and this led to the inception of the thought, that exotic animal medicine could be a strong branch of veterinary medicine, even in India. She was invited to speak about Avian Medicine in Mumbai by the Pet Practitioners Association and from here the idea, that this could be a specialization in the veterinary field seeded in the minds of veterinarians.

As mentioned earlier, there were veterinarians who were helping treat people with birds and reptiles before but it was very rare, and they were treating by chance and not by choice.

Avian Medicine in Its Infancy

Going back to the authors early days in college in the early 2000's, veterinarians serving in zoos were approached by traders who had bought these birds from abroad. Early medicine involved medication through water because neither the veterinarian nor the owner knew how to administer medication. Furthermore, for the veterinarian it was a challenge when different species of birds were presented to him/her. Professors of veterinary medicine were also presented with illness in exotic birds. It was presumed that they would have a general idea how to treat animals. However, most veterinary colleges did not have a wild or exotic animal treatment section or expertise. Therefore, they modeled the diseases from what they knew from production medicine. So, if mammals were presented they tried to find analogies with the similar species in domestic animals. From all these, birds could be modeled best because poultry medicine is quite well established in the subcontinent. Therefore, infectious diseases could be identified easily. The modality of administration, however, was not well researched and continued to be a problem. Dr. Ajit Ranade, retired Ex Dean and the author's professor of poultry medicine at the Bombay Veterinary College, was 1 such veterinarian. He was asked to treat birds that were bought to the teaching hospital. He used to prescribe medicines that he would use in poultry and had a good rate of success. (Pers Communication)

Before traveling circuses were banned in India, performing animals were also treated by zoo veterinarians, since the circuses did not have their own traveling veterinarians. Circuses had performing birds, wild animals which were non-traditional domesticated animals. From the author's personal experience, in her time as a student of veterinary medicine, she used to shadow the zoo veterinarian with the Veermata Jijabai Bhosale Udyan, commonly called as the Byculla zoo located in Mumbai. Her point of contact was, Dr. M.S. Karawale. It was through him she was introduced to the field of exotics and he was her first mentor. Due to international grain and cloth trading from South Africa, there were many 'Kasuku's '(Swahili term for gray parrot or simply parrot), which were bought by traders to Mumbai. These birds were kept as pets in trader's households for many years as the wild greys were quite resilient to disease. Prominent people used to own these birds and he used to go on house calls to treat these birds and over a period of time he would refer all these enquiriesto the author. The complaints were basic like diarrhea, trauma, fractures, and regurgitation/vomiting. To be honest, it was not a very large community and in Mumbai there may have been many more birds, however, he saw a very small number. The author remember seeing 4 to 5 regular exotic birds during her shadowing period with him, which lasted 4 years.

Reptile Medicine- Securing a Grip

Veterinarians , rarely saw reptiles at that period of time. While researching for this article, there were many similarities identified between Sri Lankan and Indian cultures, when it came to folklore about reptiles. The relationship between the Sri Lankan community and reptile fauna goes back to 10000 years when they named 1 of their ancient tribes as Nagas.[12]

Naga means snake in Sanskrit. Nagas were the native people who contributed to the formation of Sri Lanka. Sri Lanka, like India, is an agrarian country and with food grains comes rodents, with rodents come their predators, reptiles. Therefore, in almost any agricultural community there is a close relationship with reptile megafauna, for example, snakes and lizards. This is so deeply ingrained into the culture that temples sport statues of the hump nosed lizard, spectacled cobra, and crocodiles. Because of their proximity to venomous snakes, the science of snake bite treatment has originated almost 5000 years ago. The treatment in Sinhalese is called 'Sinhala Visha Vedakama.'

In the Indian culture, God's are linked with animals as their vehicles or 'vahanas' to protect them. They are also worshipped. Farmers worship the snake in a festival called 'Naag Panchami'. It falls during the time when rice is sowed in paddy fields. Folklore states that praying to the snake, more specifically the cobra, keeps farmers from being attacked by snakes and also because they recognize snakes as the protector of food grains since they keep rodents in check. There are many fascinating stories about snakes and personally, I think it is because snakes are misunderstood, feared, and revered because their behavior is not predictable by the common man.

Turtles Bring in Money!

Goddess Lakshmi, the goddess of wealth has a turtle as her vahana. Many trading organizations or even shops, commonly keep a small silver statue of a turtle submerged in water near their cash counters. The next best thing was keeping live turtles in captivity because that was better than keeping statues. In 2011 to 2012, Feng Shui made a splash India and in order to attract money, many people started keeping turtles at home.[14]

This led to a sudden boom in people keeping soft shelled and hard-shelled turtles. Lack of understanding of the biology, diet, and management of these turtles led to metabolic diseases and managemental diseases. They were and continue to be predominant in reptile medicine. Every one of India's exotic animal veterinarians is self-taught because of their interest in the subject. There is a strong dependence on texts and journals, recently journal article from the internet. We attend conferences, try to secure internships, or observer-ships to gain experience. During this time, there was a revolution among wildlife rescue and rehabbers and many new Non-Governmental Organizations (NGOs) working toward rescue and rehab arose. This is when most veterinarians with an inclination to-ward wildlife started getting hands-on experience with wildlife, which in turn translated to exotic animals. Whoever showcased an interest in non-traditional species got bombarded by the rescuers. These were the days when social media wasn't prevalent. The good old 'word of mouth' got well-meaning Samaritans to come to veterinarians for help. Along the coast, Olive Ridley turtles had been coming to India for many years. Now, they were washing up on the coast due to flipper injuries or fractures and now because the rescue trend was rampant every animal was saved. This was how a center in western Maharashtra, dedi-cated only to sea turtles, was established in a small town called Dahanu, where the chief conservator of forest was spearheading the cause. A notable name among reptile veterinarians is Dr. Dinesh Vinherkar, who worked with these stranded marine turtles. He has done a lot of good work and a picture of the prothesis flipper he created for a turtle has been published in the recent edition of Dr. Mader's text book.

BIOLOGIST AND VETERINARY ASSOCIATIONS

With NGO's sprucing up around, biologists were taking the lead and securing funds to support species specific programs around the country. One such organization was *Turtle Survival Alliance*, which the author got to interact with because of Dr. Gowri Mal-lapur. Reptile medicine is still very poorly understood in the subcontinent. Dr. Gowri Mallapur was one of the first veterinarians to immerse herself exclusively into reptile medicine in 2011. She was the head veterinarian at the Madras Crocodile Bank Trust and was the only veterinarian at the time who had a lot of information about reptile biology and links to veterinarians abroad. Together with her were initiated a program to study fresh water species in the rivers of northern and north eastern India, from a veterinary aspect. India has about 19 freshwater turtle species and there are no re-cords or vital information about their medical physiology or blood values, which we are working on and trying to publish.

Similarly, there were other programs that were started by other organizations. A very prominent one was the *Vulture Recovery Program initiated by the Bombay Natural His-tory Society (BNHS)* [14]and then adapted by the Ministry of Environment Forest and Climate Change(MOEF & CC) to the Action Plan for Vulture conservation 2020 to 2025 to prevent mortalities due to diclofenac poisoning and promote conservation breeding of this rapidly depleting species.[15] Since this was a primarily biologist led conservation action plan, and the species was critically endangered getting permis-sions to perform blood draws or procedures was a process riled with paperwork. Annual health monitoring events were organized, where veterinary experts from the United Kingdom (UK) were invited to assess the vulture's health. Bombay Natural His-tory Society set up the vulture conservation program with funding secured form the UK government through the Darwin Initiative. Veterinary guidance was provided by Dr. Nic Masters, Chief Veterinary Officer, Zoologic Society of London. Creation of vulture safe zones and provision of safe food through the Jatayu programme were auxiliary com-ponents for an effective program. Continuous advocacy for keeping meat free from diclofenac is an important part of the program, which is a work in continuum funded by small grants. There were many Indian veterinary doctors involved in the project but the most dedicated veterinarian supporting the cause is Dr. Percy Awari. He is not associated with the BNHS anymore but continues to spearhead his sole goal, saving vultures by vociferous advocacy and being a sterling member of the Saving Asians Vultures from Extinction (SAVE) group.[16] Saving Asians Vultures from

Extinction group involves all the countries from South Asia who are stakeholders in the conservation program.

WILDLIFE TRAFFIC AND EFFORTS TO CURB IT

"South Asia has been a crucial source for wildlife trafficking, as well as transit hub for illegal wildlife trade. Wildlife trafficking has been a debilitating aspect for conservation practices in South Asia.'[17] Traffickers exploit the porous borders of South Asia to smuggle wildlife products and timber within the region and beyond to other lucrative international destinations. There was a regional training to build capacity of enforcement agencies and enhance cooperation and collaboration among the countries to disrupt and deter wildlife trafficking in the region by Wildlife Institute of India and Trade Records Analysis of Flora and Fauna.

There may be laws and rules in place for trafficked wildlife, but when there are actual seizures, there are no veterinary supports and they either have to be held at the place of seizure or shipped back to the original country. (Pers comm) One Health is the mandate worldwide, but there is no surveillance performed on these trafficked animals because of an absence of exotic/wild animal veterinarians. This is a problem since no one knows under whose jurisdiction the rescued animals/birds fall. This becomes a serious issue if one has to consider transboundary or exotic diseases. Sometimes these animals may find their way into private or public animal markets. Most of these market places are controlled by the local mafia and not even the officials want to take responsibility to police them. This is the reason wildlife trade is carried out blatantly with a disregard for authority and rules. There is poor awareness about the Indian wildlife laws and the demand for exotic or Indian wildlife is supplied readily. The numbers of veterinarian with knowledge to treat these pets is very small as compared to the number of animals that need help. In South Asia alone, there are close to 100 veterinary colleges, but only a handful of schools offer wildlife medicine. The curriculum too concentrates mostly on conservation and captive breeding and doesn't have much to do with actual medicine. Disregarding a few schools, which support regional and species specific programs in the state of Kerala, where wellness checks are conducted by forests for working elephants, there is no integrated action plan to assess wildlife diseases. This is a major drawback and is something the veterinary council is working on. Currently, in the undergraduate program there is a semester on wildlife diseases and medicine, which now includes a lecture on exotic animal medicine.

INCLUSION OF EXOTIC ANIMAL MEDICINE IN THE PRIVATE PRACTICE SECTOR

The scenario in veterinary clinics has changed as regards to exotic animal medicine because there is a higher representation of exotic animal cases at veterinary clinics over the last 10 years. Birds and turtles are most represented, then come rabbits, guinea pigs, and rats. There are a few people who have the iguanas and snakes but they are not seen as much as they should be. The Ministry of Environment and Forest in 2020 started an online registration process for all exotics species to keep a check on what is being kept in captivity. The animals that were not registered were confiscated or heavy fines were levied. The portal to register is called PARIVESH and one of its roles is to declare and in a way document exotic animal ownership. Some other things this web-based application does are submission and monitoring proposals seeking environment, forest, wildlife, and cosatal regulation zone clearances from the central, state, and district level authorthies.The Wildlife Act was amended to include lesser known species and to raise the bar for all commonly found animals kept in captivity, which people used to keep since they were Schedule 3 or 4 animals, to a schedule which would be punishable by law.

THE WAY FORWARD

To sum it up, exotic animal medicine is a rapidly evolving field in the subcontinent. Great efforts are being taking to increase active and passive surveillance for disease monitoring. Regulation of exotic animal trade is also being looked into. The veterinary schools are warming up to the idea to have specialty programs, where this branch of medicine can be taught. The number of veterinarians with an interest in exotics has increased and there are many more clinics that see exotic animals in the country because the interest is piqued. We have our own small conferences, where leading international speakers are invited to speak on topics pertinent to exotics. The number of exotic species is increasing, however, not everyone is sure if it is because of more trafficking or better breeding facilities. The future of this branch of science looks bright. Let us hope the conservation efforts also pay off.

Note: The latter part of the manuscript has been compiled after speaking with veterinarians whose names have been mentioned in the document and from personal experience. These were one of the forerunners of exotic animal medicine in the country.

CLINICS CARE POINTS

- Referrals from other veterinarians.
- Continuing education or expertise aquired over a period of time by the veterinarian.
- Facilites available to treat exotics in practice.
- Understanding the biology of the species they were treating.
- Ability to perform surgical or medical interventions even when they were financially or technologicallly challenged.
- Emergency and critical care services.

DISCLOSURE

The author declares that she has no relevant or material financial interests that relate to the research described in this paper.

REFERENCES

1. Rahman SA. The history of veterinary medicine in India. AAVMC 2004. Available at: https://jvme.utpjournals.press/doi/pdf/10.3138/jvme.31.1.55/. [Accessed 14 January 2024].
2. Chakraborty S. History of animal keeping in ancient india and its socio-economic. Scientific Applicability in 21st century 2023;6–10. https://doi.org/10.32996/pbjpsh.
3. Brown WN, Edgerton F. The Elephant-Lore of the Hindus. J Am Orient Soc 1932; 52(1):89.
4. Sahu BP. Patterns of animal use in ancient India. Available at: Proceedings of the Indian History Congress 1932;48:66–75 https://www.jstor.org/Stable/44141651.

5. History of veterinary medicine in India. Available at: http://ecoursesonline.iasri. res.in/mod/page/view.php?id=70072/. [Accessed 14 January 2024].

6. Mazumdar GP, Banerjee SC. The asiatic society. Avaiable at: https://archive.org/ download/Bibliotheca_Indica_Series/KrishiParasara.

7. Shamshatra. kautilya arthashastra. Available at: https://csboa.in/eBooks/Artha shastra_of_Chanakya_-_English.pdf.

8. Rastogi S, Kaphle K. Sustainable traditional medicine: taking the inspirations from ancient veterinary science. Evid base Compl Alternative Med 2011;1–6. https:// doi.org/10.1093/ecam/nen071.

9. 16th Century bird dispensary in Khambat to get a modern facelift. Available at: https://timesofindia.indiatimes.com/city/vadodara/16th-century-bird-dispensary-in-khambhat-to-get-modern-facelift/articleshow/80076623.cms. [Accessed 26 December 2023].

10. Available at: https://www.getbengal.com/details/asias-first-zoo-at-barrackpore-was-even-older-to-london-zoo-surprised. [Accessed 29 December 2023].

11. Walker. Major events and trends in Indian zoo since independence with particular reference to the national zoo policy, 1998. Zoos' Print 1999;XIV:3–10.

12. Gunathilaka T., Agalawatta W. and Bandara C., Sense of community ; local peoples perception on reptile with cultural aspect of conservation . a case study in Sri Lanka, 2012, Natural Science Foundation. Available at: https://www. researchgate.net/publication/271767248_SENSE_OF_COMMUNITY_LOCAL_ PEOPLE'S_PERCEPTION_ON_REPTILES_WITH_CULTURAL_ASPECT_ON_ CONSERVATIONA_CASE_STUDY_IN_SRI_LANKA.

13. The wildlife (protection) Act. 1972. Available at: https://www.indiacode.nic.in/ bitstream/123456789/1726/1/a1972-53.pdf.

14. Available at: https://timesofindia.indiatimes.com/city/ahmedabad/illegal-turtle-trade-unabated-in-ahmedabad/articleshow/15524589.cms.

15. Available at: https://www.bnhs.org/public/pdf_documents/1562761806.pdf.

16. Saving vultures from extinction – policy brief. Aviailable at: https://save-vultures. org/wp-content/uploads/2020/02/Vulture-policy-brief-India-Feb-20-updated-3.pdf.

17. South Asian countries meet again to strengthen efforts to curb Widlife trafficking. Available at: https://www.wwfindia.org/?26802/south-asian-countries-meet-again-to-strengthen-efforts-to-curb-wildlife-trafficking.

Exotic Animal Practice in Africa

Johannes Lodewicus Coetzee de Beer, BVSc (Hons), MANZCVS (Avian Health)

KEYWORDS

• Avian • Exotic practice • Africa • Challenges • Common species

KEY POINTS

• Historical evolution:

Exotic animal practice in South Africa had a slower start compared to international counterparts.

Dedicated exotic practices emerged slowly, initially serviced by general practice veterinarians or those with a special interest in avian and exotic medicine.

• Interesting aspects of avian and exotic medicine practice:

A wide variety of exotic species, including avian, reptile, and unique wildlife, challenging veterinarians to broaden their knowledge.

Caseload diversity creates ample opportunities for research, as Africa likely harbors undiscovered pathogens.

Infancy of exotic animal practice in South Africa offers opportunities to establish primary facilities.

Continued

INTRODUCTION

In South Africa, exotic animal practice had a slower start compared to our international counterparts (**Table 1**). The popularity of exotic pets preceded the establishment of sole exotic practices. Initially, these patients were attended to either by their local general practice veterinarian or by those with a special interest in avian and exotic medicine. These special interest veterinarians would have to travel from town to town due to the large land area and relatively sparse veterinary coverage for these species. They would perform surgical sexing along with consultation and treatment of companion avian and exotic patients where they could locally; however, this presented challenges as they did not always have the necessary equipment on hand for comprehensive diagnostics and lacked facilities for admission for treatment. Consequently, patients would receive less than gold-standard care and patients were sometimes left in the care of laypeople while the attending veterinarians moved on to their next location.

Pellmeadow Estate, Klapmuts, South Africa
E-mail address: coetzee@birdclinic.co.za

Vet Clin Exot Anim 27 (2024) 561–571
https://doi.org/10.1016/j.cvex.2024.03.009
1094-9194/24/© 2024 Elsevier Inc. All rights reserved.

vetexotic.theclinics.com

Continued

- Specific challenges:

  Limited education infrastructure and emphasis on exotic animal practice in core curricula.

  Challenges in nutritional control due to unregulated feeds and poor-quality seed mixes.

  Increasing use of herbal medicine without scientific evidence and potential adverse effects.

  Client education challenges due to the scarcity of dedicated practices.

  Limited diagnostic resources, disease outbreaks (eg, rabbit hemorrhagic disease virus [RHDV]), and power supply disruptions.

  Load shedding, a common practice due to power grid limitations, adversely affects veterinary practices.

- Diseases and regulatory response:

  RHDV outbreak presented significant challenges, emphasizing the need for proactive measures.

  Limited availability of internationally recognized medications and overzealous use of medications, contributing to antibiotic resistance.

- Future trajectory:

  Establishing affiliations with international associations to elevate standards.

  Inclusion of specialized courses on exotic animals in education.

  Stricter regulations for nutritional control.

  Advocacy, collaboration, and innovation to address diagnostic challenges and financial hurdles.

This started to change in the 1980s, however, with the opening of the first dedicated avian practice as the popularity of exotic species increased. Dedicated practices became more common in the 2000s, although not to the extent seen in other countries. Most of these veterinarians were self-taught, and only a handful spent time with international specialists. The situation is improving somewhat in this regard, however, with the presence of a small number of internationally trained or experienced veterinarians delivering care from dedicated avian and exotic practices.

WHAT MAKES SOUTH AFRICA UNIQUE?

South Africa's unique veterinary landscape is shaped by the varied climates spanning its 9 provinces. In KwaZulu-Natal,[1] the tropical climate prevails, creating an environment suitable for a diverse range of fauna compared to the arid expanses of the Karoo,[2] with challenges posed by extreme temperatures and scarce water resources. The Western Cape[3] introduces a temperate climate, marked by milder conditions.

These climate nuances significantly impact the species inhabiting each region. The rock hyrax and meerkat, accustomed to semiarid and arid environments, contrasts with the vervet monkey and bushbaby, thriving in tropical landscapes.

Understanding these climatic differences is pivotal for veterinarians, as it directly influences the health and well-being of exotic animals under their care. Moreover, such diversity underscores the need for adaptable veterinary practices tailored to the specific challenges posed by each region's climate and the unique species it supports.

Table 1
This is an example of a medicine box provided to aviculturists. This is unfortunately very common and poses massive risks

Trade name	Active Ingredient	Dosage	Comment
Antibiotics			
Baytril 5% injection	Enrofloxacin 50 mg/mL	0.02 mL/100 g once daily (SID)	—
Enrovet 10%	Enrofloxacin 100 mg/mL	0.01 mL/100 g SID 1 mL/500 mL water	—
Amikacin 250 mg/2 mL	Amikacin 250 mg/2 mL	0.01 mL/100 g BID	Protect kidneys
Nuflor injection	Florfenicol 300 mg/mL	0.01 mL/150 g every 48 h	—
Clamentin-S	Amoxicillin 25 mg/mL + clavulanic acid 6.35 mg/mL	0.1 mL/100 g BID	Reconstitute as indicated
Synulox 50 mg tab	Amoxicillin 40 mg + clavulanic acid 10 mg	1 tab/2500 g BID 1/4 tab/625 g BID	—
Psittavet injection	Doxycycline HCl 50 mg/mL	0.1 mL/100 g every 5 d	—
Doxybiotic-Plus	Doxycycline HCl 75 g/kg + Vit A, B1, B2, B6, B12, E, K, lactose, and dextrose	5 g/L water or 1 g/3 kg birds in soft food	Doxycycline binds calcium
Supadox 50	Doxycycline HCl 541 g/kg	1 g/20 kg birds in soft food	—
Flagyl oral suspension	Metronidazole 40 mg/mL	0.05 mL/100 g BID	—
Antifungals			
Nystatin oral	Nystasin 100,000 IU/mL	0.1 mL/100 g BID	First day TID
Itraconazole 5 mg	Itraconazole 5 mg	1 cap/kg BID	—
VFend 50 mg	Voriconazole 5 mg	1/4 tab/kg BID	—
VFend 40 mg/mL	Voriconazole 40 mg/mL	0.03/100 g BID	—
Fluconazole	Fluconazole 150 mg	5 mg/kg SID	—
Anti-inflammatory			
Metacam injection	Meloxicam 20 mg/mL	0.01 mL/200–400 g SID	—
Petcam	Meloxicam 5 mg/mL	0.05 mL/100 g SID	—
Finadyne	Flunixin meglumine 50 mg/mL	0.01 g/100 g SID	—
Dexa 0.2/Kortico	Dexamethazone 2 mg/mL	0.1 mg/100 g SID	—

WHAT MAKES AVIAN AND EXOTIC MEDICINE PRACTICE IN SOUTH AFRICA INTERESTING?

Due to South Africa's unique landscape and challenges, a wide variety of species present to exotic animal practices, encompassing diverse avian, reptile, and other wildlife species unique to Africa. This diversity provides veterinarians with challenges rarely seen in other parts of the world and encourages them to broaden their knowledge and invest in their professional development. The hugely variable anatomy and physiology of the species presenting, coupled with uncommon disease processes and pathogens, creates an incredibly stimulating work environment for any practitioner. Not only does this provide for engaging day-to-day practice but also it creates ample opportunities for research and development into evolving or, as yet, undiscovered pathogens and diseases. For this reason, exotic animal medicine in Africa is an excellent environment for any practitioner from around the world to further develop their knowledge and skills. This coupled with the infancy of exotic animal practice in South Africa brings exciting opportunities to establish new primary facilities, expand available services, and continue to improve the care provided to exotic species in this part of the globe.

COMMONLY SEEN EXOTIC AVIAN SPECIES

Africa (South Africa):
- Orange-winged amazon
  (*Amazona amazonica*)
- Gray parrot
  (*Psittacus erithacus*)
- Cockatiel
  (*Nymphicus hollandicus*)
- Budgerigar
  (*Melopsittacus undulatus*)
- Ring-necked parakeet
  (*Psittacula krameri*)
- Peach-faced lovebird
  (*Agapornis roseicollis*)
- Chicken
  (*Gallus gallus domesticus*)
- Canary
  (*Serinus canaria domestica*)
- Eclectus parrot
  (*Eclectus roratus*)
- Pyrrhura conure sp
- Chicken
  (*G gallus domesticus*)
- Lorikeets
  (tribe Loriini)
- Pigeons and doves
  (Order: Columbiformes,
  Family: Columbidae)
- Blue and gold macaw
  (*Ara ararauna*)
- Scarlet macaw
  (*Ara macao*)

Green-winged macaw
(Ara chloropterus)
Ring-necked parakeet
(P krameri)
Mealy Amazon
(Amazona farinosa)
Senegal parrot
(Poicephalus senegalus)
Umbrella cockatoo
(Cacatua alba)
Rose-breasted cockatoo
(Eolophus roseicapilla)
Sun conure
(Aratinga solstitialis)
Yellow-crowned Amazon
(Amazona ochrocephala)
Blue-fronted Amazon
(Amazona aestiva)
Alexandrine parakeet
(Psittacula eupatria)
Blue-headed pionus
(Pionus menstruus)
Commonly seen exotic small mammal species:
Rabbit (Lagomorph)
Guinea pig (Cavia porcellus)
Ferret (Mustela putorius furo)
Capuchin (Cebinae)
Marmoset (Callithrix sp)
Chinchilla (Chinchilla sp)
Commonly seen exotic reptile species:
Python species (Pythonidae)
Boa species
Iguana species (Pogona sp)
Bearded dragon species

WHAT SPECIFIC CHALLENGES DOES AVIAN AND EXOTIC PRACTICE FACE IN SOUTH AFRICA?
Limited University and Education Infrastructure

Being an exotic veterinarian in Africa is challenging due to the limited number of universities offering relevant programs. In South Africa, where only The University of Pretoria provides a veterinary program, the scarcity of institutions matched with an increasing demand puts pressure on the available resources and faculty. The challenges are exacerbated by financial constraints, affecting the quality of education and resources available for aspiring exotic veterinarians.

Exotic Animal Practice Not Emphasized in Core Curriculum

The lack of emphasis on exotic animal practice in the core veterinary curriculum adds another layer of difficulty. Elective courses frequently offer only a handful of lectures on exotic animals, leaving graduates with limited exposure to this specialized field. Comparative anatomy, for instance, might focus primarily on common animals like chickens, rather than a broader range of exotic species. Additionally, only a small number have international experience, further limiting the exchange of knowledge and best practices in exotic animal care.

Unregulated Avian Feeds and Poor-quality Seed Mixes

The prevalence of unregulated feeds in exotic animal diets poses a multifaceted challenge for veterinarians. With the sale of unregistered feeds lacking standardized quality control and appropriate nutritional breadth, multiple nutritional deficiencies add complexity to determining the cause of presenting disease. Veterinary communities, often small, share cases related to specific products, necessitating substantial financial investments in evaluating these feeds as a potential contributing factor to ill health.

The absence of regulatory oversight not only compromises the nutritional integrity of these feeds but also increases the risk of contamination and subsequent infectious disease in addition to nutrient deficiency. These poor-quality feeds frequently result in severe bacterial and fungal airsacculitis, while nutritional deficiencies, such as hypervitaminosis A, hepatic and cardiac diseases, hypocalcemic-related presentations, and obesity-related diseases, become prevalent. Addressing this issue requires a push for quality control measures in the production of avian diets and enhanced education on proper avian nutrition to mitigate the health risks associated with inadequate seed mixes.

Lagomorph Diets and Local Feeds

Nutritional issues are not isolated to the avian population. Lagomorphs frequently face dietary challenges due to the cost and limited availability of international brands. Naive clients may opt for locally available alternatives, such as equine pellets, which do not meet the specific nutritional needs of these animals. This dietary choice can lead to a range of health issues, including dental problems, gastrointestinal complications, and obesity-related diseases. Addressing this challenge involves promoting awareness about species-specific diets, even when faced with economic constraints.

Herbal Medicine

The increasing use of herbal medicine introduces complexities, especially when these herbs are sold by traditional medicine practitioners lacking qualifications in conventional medicine and nutrition. The absence of scientific evidence supporting herbal remedies and the limited understanding of potential adverse effects create uncertainties for veterinarians. The challenge of identifying specific herbs responsible for diseases is amplified due to the diverse array included in herbal mixes, emphasizing the need for evidence-based practices and education in herbal medicine use. The following are just some of the substances included in some preparations.

African green clay (Montmorillonite clay)
African potato (*Hypoxis hemerocallidea*)
Agrimony (*Agrimonia* spp)
Alfalfa (*Medicago sativa*)
Aloe vera (*Aloe barbadensis miller*)
Aniseed (*Pimpinella anisum*)
Arnica oil extracts (*Arnica montana*)
Ashwagandha (*Withania somnifera*)
Astragalus (*Astragalus* spp)
Bearberry (*Arctostaphylos uva-ursi*)
Bilberry (*Vaccinium myrtillus*)

Black cohosh (*Actaea racemosa*)
Black seed (*Nigella sativa*)
Black walnut (*Juglans nigra*)
Borage (*Borago officinalis*)
Boswellia (*Boswellia serrata*)
Bromelain (Pineapple enzyme)
Buchu (*Agathosma* spp)
Burdock (*Arctium lappa*)
Calendula (*Calendula officinalis*)
Cancer bush (*Sutherlandia frutescens*)
Castor oil (*Ricinus communis*)
Catnip (*Nepeta cataria*)
Cat's claw (*Uncaria tomentosa*)
Centella (*Centella asiatica*)
Chamomile (*Matricaria chamomilla*)
Chaste berries (*Vitex agnus-castus*)
Chickweed (*Stellaria media*)
Clove (*Syzygium aromaticum*)
Coconut oil (*Cocos nucifera*)
Comfrey (*Symphytum officinale*)
Copaiba essential oils (*Copaifera* spp)
Curcumin (*Curcuma longa*)
Devil's claw (*Harpagophytum procumbens*)
Echinacea (*Echinacea* spp)
Elderberries (*Sambucus* spp)
Elecampane (*Inula helenium*)
Frankincense oleoresins (*Boswellia* spp)
Gentian (*Gentiana* spp)
Golden seal (*Hydrastis canadensis*)
Hawthorn berries (*Crataegus* spp)
Hemp seed oil (*Cannabis sativa*)
Hops (*Humulus lupulus*)
Horehound (*Marrubium vulgare*)
Horsetail (*Equisetum arvense*)
Juniper berries (*Juniperus communis*)
Kelp (*Laminaria* spp)
Lady's mantle (*Alchemilla* spp)
Lavender essential oil (*Lavandula* spp)
Lemon balm (*Melissa officinalis*)
Lemongrass (*Cymbopogon citratus*)
Licorice root (*Glycyrrhiza glabra*)
Maca (*Lepidium meyenii*)
Marigold (*C officinalis*)
Marshmallow (*Althaea officinalis*)
Meadowsweet (*Filipendula ulmaria*)
Mullein flowers (*Verbascum* spp)
Moringa (*Moringa oleifera*)
Motherwort (*Leonurus cardiaca*)
Myrrh (*Commiphora* spp)
Neem leaves (*Azadirachta indica*)
Neem oil (*A indica*)

Nettle (*Urtica dioica*)
Oat (*Avena sativa*)
Olive leaf (*Olea europaea*)
Olive oil (*O europaea*)
Pau d'Arco (*Tabebuia impetiginosa*)
Peppermint (*Mentha piperita*)
Quassia (*Quassia* spp)
Raspberry leaf (*Rubus idaeus*)
Red clover (*Trifolium pratense*)
Rhodiola (*Rhodiola rosea*)
Rose essential oil (*Rosa* spp)
Rose hydrosol (*Rosa* spp)
Sage (*Salvia officinalis*)
Saw palmetto (*Serenoa repens*)
Schisandra (*Schisandra chinensis*)
Seaweed (Various species)
Skullcap (*Scutellaria* spp)
Slippery elm (*Ulmus rubra*)
Sodium bicarbonate: $NaHCO_3$
Sodium carbonate: Na_2CO_3
Sodium hypochlorite (to soak sprouts): $NaClO$
Spirulina (*Arthrospira* spp)
St John's wort (*Hypericum perforatum*)
Stinging nettle (*U dioica*)
Sweet almond oil (*Prunus dulcis*)
Tea tree oil (*Melaleuca alternifolia*)
Valerian (*Valeriana officinalis*)
Vegetable glycerine: Glycerol
Witch hazel (*Hamamelis virginiana*)
Wormwood (*Artemisia absinthium*)
Yarrow (*Achillea millefolium*)

Client Education

The importance of client education is emphasized due to the lack of exotic animal practices and the large pet-owning population. Bridging the knowledge gap is crucial for empowering pet owners to make informed decisions about the nutrition and care of their exotic animals. Overcoming client education challenges involves expanding access to information, fostering communication between veterinarians and clients, and emphasizing the significance of proper care practices for the well-being of exotic species.

Limited Diagnostic Resources

As a third-world country, the scarcity of advanced diagnostic tools poses a significant challenge for veterinarians. While some practices have gained access to computed tomography, the prohibitive costs hinder widespread use. This limitation is particularly problematic for accurately diagnosing dental issues and otitis media in rabbits, where precise imaging is crucial for an effective treatment planning. The absence of other investigations like modern polymerase chain reaction (PCR) diagnostics for certain exotic animal diseases, such as Avian Bornavirus or reptile viruses, also falls short of international standards. Additionally, testing for conditions like *Encephalitozoon cuniculi* is constrained to postmortem or renal histopathology, limiting real-time diagnostics and timely intervention.

Even where testing is available, priority is often given to production, equine, and other companion animals ahead of avian and exotic samples. All of this is compounded by a shortage of pathologists experienced in exotic animal practice. This combination of factors presents avian and exotic veterinarians with significant challenges in preventing, managing, and treating diseases across our patient population.

Specific Diseases and Regulatory Response

Rabbit hemorrhagic disease virus (RHDV) has presented a significant challenge in South Africa. The ban on Lagomorph importation, driven by concerns for the critically endangered Riverine rabbit, did not prevent the widespread deaths of Lagomorphs in 2022. It took several months, involving postmortems, PCRs, and serotyping, to identify RHDV serotype 2 as the causative agent due to communication gaps and limited resources.

The response to RHDV included an emergency permit application for an unregistered vaccine, a process that consumed 5 months, making the vaccine available only in May 2023. Unfortunately, due to naivety and a delayed response from authorities, the disease spread across the country, highlighting the need for more proactive measures.

Logistical Issues

Load shedding is a concept that many outside Africa will not be familiar with. Due to years of underinvestment and reported corruption, the power grids do not have capacity to maintain supply 24 hours a day. As a result, scheduled power cuts for up to 14 hours a day are a reality in South Africa and some other African countries. This clearly adversely affects veterinary practices, limiting access to lighting, essential equipment, disrupting the cold chain and impacting patient care, especially for reptiles and chinchillas vulnerable to temperature fluctuations.

Limited Medication Availability or Inappropriate Medication Use

The overzealous use of medications is a widespread issue globally, exacerbated by a lack of knowledge in certain regions. Antibiotic resistance is prevalent, as evidenced in culture and sensitivity reports. In some cases, individuals, particularly in aviculture, supply medications without proper understanding, resulting in microbe resistance, partially treated or even exacerbated conditions, or unintended complications. Unfortunately, this happens when traveling veterinarians supply aviculturists with these boxes without seeing the patient or conducting diagnostics. This issue has been brought to the attention of the South African Veterinary Council, yet there has been no response or intervention. An example medication box supplied to some breeders is shown in the later discussion.

Outside of avian medicine, Lagomorph sinusitis/rhinitis, for example, often receives prolonged broad-spectrum antibiotic treatment without proper diagnostics, leading to resistant strains. This emphasizes the importance of informed and targeted medical approaches to avoid escalating problems.

The lack of internationally available medications is also a recurring issue, with common drugs like buprenorphine and amphotericin B remaining elusive for an extended period. This can lead to the inappropriate use of other medications, further adding to the issue of resistance.

Continuing Professional Development

Continuing professional development is important for any practitioner but even more so for those practicing in a specialist field in small or single-handed practices. Seeing learned and experienced colleagues practicing and discussing cases is the corner-stone of ensuring your practice is up to date with the current general consensus. In a country with very few avian and exotic veterinarians, and where they are often hundreds or thousands of kilometers apart, this poses considerable challenges. With modern technology, it is easier to communicate, discuss cases, share imaging, and consult each other for a collegiate opinion. Access to international conferences and ongoing learning remains important, however, and can prove financially very difficult for individual practitioners given these are usually held in Europe, North America, or Australasia.

FUTURE TRAJECTORY

For avian and exotic animal practice in South Africa to flourish, there needs to be a concerted effort to elevate its standards to match those of our international counter-parts. An imperative first step would involve establishing a dedicated committee or branch affiliated with esteemed international associations such as The Association of Avian Veterinarians, The Association of Exotic Mammal Veterinarians, and The Association of Reptile Amphibian Veterinarians. This strategic move would open doors for South African veterinarians to access global insights, best practices, and ongoing research in the field of exotic animal medicine.

To fortify the foundation of knowledge among veterinary professionals, a push for the inclusion of specialized courses focusing on exotic animals is paramount. These courses should cover a spectrum of essential topics, including anatomy, physiology, husbandry, and common diseases. By providing such comprehensive education, we empower general practitioners with the fundamental understanding required to deliver optimal care for the diverse array of species encountered in exotic animal practice. While recognizing the importance of public education in promoting responsible exotic pet ownership, we must acknowledge the challenges presented by socioeconomic disparities. Efforts to disseminate information should be tailored to different demographics, utilizing diverse communication channels to ensure a broad reach and impact.

The critical issue of nutritional control demands attention, particularly concerning food products available to the general public. Stricter regulations would ideally ensure that patients receive the necessary nutritional requirements, thereby mitigating the risk of metabolic and related diseases. However, the unfortunate reality of corruption in many African countries complicates the implementation of such controls, necessi-tating advocacy and collaborative efforts to address systemic issues.

In the face of challenges related to diagnostics, commonly used drugs, and the financial hurdles associated with establishing a practice, the veterinary community must embark on an exploration of alternative methods. Innovation becomes impera-tive in this context. Collaborating with academic institutions and securing research grants can facilitate the development and implementation of cutting-edge diagnostic tools and therapeutic approaches, allowing veterinarians to adapt and excel despite resource constraints.

In essence, this holistic and proactive approach, encompassing education, collab-oration, and innovation, lays the groundwork for a future where exotic animal practice in South Africa stands on par with international standards, ensuring the well-being of both practitioners and the diverse range of species under their care.

SUMMARY

The development of exotic animal practice in South Africa has been slow compared to global standards, facing challenges such as limited education infrastructure, lack of emphasis on exotic animals in core curricula, the lack of availability of international standard testing and treatments, and the challenges posed by crumbling national infrastructure. The future requires a concerted effort, including specialized education, public awareness, stricter regulations, and innovative approaches to elevate the standards of exotic animal practice in South Africa.

DISCLOSURE

The author has nothing to disclose.

REFERENCES

1. Ndlovu MS, Demlie M. Assessment of meteorological drought and wet conditions using two drought indices across kwazulu-natal province, South Africa. Atmosphere 2020;11(6):623.
2. Bradshaw PL, Cowling RM. Landscapes, rock types, and climate of the Greater Cape Floristic Region. In: Allsopp N, Colville JF, Anthony, editors. Verboom G., *Fynbos: ecology, evolution, and conservation of a megadiverse region*, online edn. Oxford: Oxford Academic; 2014. p. 26–46.
3. Botai CM, Botai JO, De Wit JP, et al. Drought characteristics over the Western Cape Province, South Africa. Water 2017;9(11):876.

Exotic Animal Practice in Europe

Daniel Calvo Carrasco, LV, CertAVP(ZM), DipECZM(Avian), MRCVS[a,*]

KEYWORDS

• Exotic pet practice • Europe • Brexit • Cascade

KEY POINTS

• Exotic pet medicine in Europe encompasses a wide range of nondomesticated animals, with diverse perceptions among veterinary professionals and the public.
• Brexit has introduced regulatory challenges, supply chain disruptions, and workforce issues, impacting exotic veterinary practices in the UK.
• Legislation changes in European countries aim to regulate exotic pet keeping, adopting positive and negative list approaches with a focus on environmental concerns.
• Veterinary medication regulations, including the EU's Regulation (EU) 2019/6, play a role in harmonizing standards and addressing the use of off-license medications in exotic practice.
• The COVID-19 pandemic and the cost-of-living crisis have influenced pet ownership trends, increased demand for veterinary services, and highlighted challenges in workforce management.

INTRODUCTION

This article differs from previous issues, as it focusses on a nonclinical, although very relevant, topic, overviewing the current situation in this field of work. Exotic practice is a clearly understood concept, but not necessarily as clearly defined, with multiple sections of our scope of work overlapping with other fields within veterinary medicine.

This article is also intended to be evidence based, and present facts, but it will also differ from other issues on the amount of type of references used.

It is not within the scope of this article to clearly define concepts, but the clarification of terms covered in the article will help to identify and understand the areas of discussion. The references or sources used, as well as the understanding of concepts will be retrieved (when available) from European sources, which might differ from other geographic locations.

a Veterinary Healthcare, Mandai Wildlife Group, Singapore
* Corresponding author.
E-mail address: Danicalvocarrasco@gmail.com

Vet Clin Exot Anim 27 (2024) 573–583
https://doi.org/10.1016/j.cvex.2024.03.010
1094-9194/24/© 2024 Elsevier Inc. All rights reserved.

vetexotic.theclinics.com

Exotic Pet is a term used widely in the English-speaking countries to refer to those animals kept as pets, which are nondomesticated animals, and will include both native and nonnative species.[1] However, one of the most seen species, and most likely the most common species seen in treated in exotic pet practice, is the domestic rabbit, *Oryctolagus cuniculus* subsp. *Domesticus*, despite being domesticated for centuries,[2] and captive bred for more than 2000 years.[2,6] Indeed, this reflects statistics that report rabbits as the 3rd most commonly kept animal as pet[7], at least in the UK. The perception of them being "exotic" pets is not consistent across veterinary professionals, nor is it consistent with the general public, with many clients being confused when a referral to an "exotic specialist" is suggested by a first opinion veterinarian (or general practitioner) suggests more specialized veterinary care.

In the French speaking community, and to a lesser degree also in other Latin languages, the term "New Companion animals" is commonly used ("Nouveaux Animaux de Compagnie" in French[3,4] o "Nuevos Animales de Compañía" in Spanish[5] often abbreviated as "NAC" in both languages, but an extremely popular term in the French speaking community). This term could be considered by some to be a better fit, as the term "Exotic" is often associated with or linked to nonnative species. Some of the species that end up being treated by exotic clinicians or exotic practices, include, to a different extent, animals kept by zoologic institutions, wildlife, farm animals, confiscated animals (intended for the pet trade or not) and stowaway animals, on top of those animals clearly kept as pets; as a discipline, Zoologic Medicine seems to be a more accurate term. In the author's opinion, trying to clearly define the species or scenarios ranges is often an unproductive exercise, and it is easier to define what is not an exotic pet instead: domestic Small animals, horses and farm animals. In practical terms, the exotic clinicians practicing in Europe are, in the majority of cases, willing to treat any animal presented to them not commonly seen by other veterinary professionals.

Exotic pet medicine is practice in both general practice or companion animal practiced, as well as in more specialized set ups.[8] Exotic pets have been treated in veterinary facilities for as long as any other species, with evidence of falconry birds being treated in Europe centuries ago.[9] The concept of modern veterinary practices providing care to pet animals is a relatively new concept with one of the oldest known practice dating from 1813.[10] At the time, most universities whereby focused on the care of horses and farm animals, following the trend initiated by the first veterinary school in France[11]; most likely, the professionals at the time would have treated any presented animal in need.

It is not possible to established when the first practice exclusively dedicated to exotics appeared in Europe, especially as many might not have originated as exotic practices. Exotic Practices might have appeared, earlier, but started to popularize from the early to mid 90's in western European countries.

It is also difficult to establish which percentage of the exotic pets seen by veterinarians in Europe are seen in exotic practices, compared with general practice; most likely, a larger proportion of exotic pets are still seen in general practice compared with exotic practice. Many factors could play a role in this, but that discussion is not within the scope of this article. A search on the Royal College of Veterinary Surgeons (RCVS) Website, the regulatory body of veterinary activities, allows to look for practice according to the species they see. A total of 1981 veterinary practices were found treating exotic/wild animal.[12] Furthermore, a search on the veterinarians' members of exotic related veterinary associations was made at the same time.

The Association of Exotic Mammal Veterinarians (AEMV)[13] had 31 veterinarians registered within the UK; the European Association of Avian Veterinarians (EAAV) website does not have the feature "Find a Vet," so the Association of Avian Veterinarians was used instead (AAV).[14] The search reported 25 veterinarians.

Last, the Association of Reptile and Amphibian Veterinarians (ARAV) has 21 veterinarians registered within the UK. It is worth noticing that some of the registered veterinarians were found in all of the 3 associations, and not all of the colleagues found work in veterinary practice (as some work in Zoologic institutions, wildlife rehabilitation centers, conservation organizations, regulatory bodies...academia). There is... is a big discrepancy at least between practices seeing exotics in the UK and veterinarians registered in at least one of the association of veterinarians of exotic mammals, reptiles, amphibians and birds. Veterinarians with a special interest, or postgraduate qualifications in the field, are those likely to be focusing in their area of interest, practicing in more dedicated or target practices.

Other European countries might not have the exact same situation as the UK and might differ in significant aspects. The UK is one of the leading countries in the veterinary field within Europe and has benefit until recently from the talent of the neighboring countries. A survey that including colleagues from 30 European countries did not explicitly state the percentage of veterinarians working in exotic-only practice versus general practice. However, it did mention that 71.8% of the respondents work mainly in companion animal practice, 12.57% mainly with food-producing animals, 3.1% in equine practice, and 12% specifically with zoo or exotic animals.

Despite being an area of increasing interest, the exotic veterinary practice remains, overall, still a relatively small portion of the overall veterinary activity in European Countries, and most of the exotic pet medicine occurs in first opinion practices.

RECENT CHANGES/CHALLENGES
Brexit

The decision by the United Kingdom to depart from the European Union, colloquially known as Brexit, has had far-reaching implications across various sectors, which has obviously also impacted the veterinary industry as a whole, and the field of exotic veterinary practice is no exception. Brexit has had a direct impact in many different areas. One of the significant impacts of Brexit on exotic veterinary practice lies in the realm of regulation. Prior to Brexit, veterinarians in the UK adhered to EU-wide regulations governing the import and export of animals, including exotic species. With the departure from the EU, the UK has gained more autonomy in setting its regulatory framework. Leaving the EU and most importantly, the EU single market, directly implies the need for regulation, and therefore paperwork, for both goods (including animals, and veterinary supplies of all sorts) and its citizens, who were able to move freely prior to this. While this independence may present opportunities for tailored regulations, it also introduces challenges, such as potential misalignment with EU standards, which still remain their main trade partner. Exotic veterinary practitioners now face the task of navigating a more complex regulatory landscape, adapting to new licensing requirements, and ensuring compliance with evolving standards.

Brexit has triggered disruptions in the supply chain of veterinary medicines and specialized equipment essential for exotic animal care. The increased bureaucracy associated with new border controls and customs procedures has led to delays in the importation of crucial supplies. Exotic veterinary practices are grappling with the consequences of these disruptions, including shortages of medications and diagnostic tools. This has not only posed challenges to the timely treatment of exotic animals but also increased the financial burden on veterinary practices as they seek alternative sources and absorb higher costs.

The veterinary profession relies heavily on international collaboration and the exchange of expertise. Brexit has created uncertainties for the mobility of veterinary professionals, potentially affecting the recruitment and retention of skilled exotic veterinarians. The end of free movement between the UK and the EU has made it more cumbersome for veterinary professionals from EU countries to work in the UK and vice versa. This may lead to a talent drain, limiting the diversity of skills and experiences available in the exotic veterinary sector.

The economic fallout from Brexit has implications for both veterinary practices and pet owners. Economic uncertainties have led to changes in consumer behavior, potentially affecting the demand for exotic pets and veterinary services. Moreover, the overall economic climate may influence the financial resources available to pet owners for veterinary care, impacting the revenue streams of exotic veterinary practices.

In conclusion, Brexit has brought about a series of challenges for the exotic veterinary practice in the UK. From regulatory changes and supply chain disruptions to workforce challenges and economic impacts, the sector is navigating uncharted territory. As the industry adapts to these changes, collaboration between veterinary professionals, regulatory bodies, and policymakers will be crucial in ensuring the continued well-being of exotic animals and the sustainability of the exotic veterinary profession in the post-Brexit era.

Legislation changes: regulation of exotic pets

In the last few years, many European countries have started to regulate exotic pet keeping. The regulatory landscape surrounding exotic pets in European countries is not only characterized by diverse approaches to ownership but also incorporates measures to address the potential threat of invasive species. In some countries, the legislation is still being discussed, in other countries, implementation has not occurred yet, and in a few, the legislation has been implemented for years. The laws and sensitivities have been as diverse as Europe itself, but two main approaches have appeared. Most of the laws regulating this in the different European countries are relatively recent, and their impacts on the long term are unknown. It is possible that some of the pet trade previously done legally might be transferred to the illegal trade; The European Union is one of the most important markets for the trafficking of endangered species and a major transit point for illegal wildlife trade.[15] It remains to be seen if the prohibition of keeping exotic pets will truly reduce the numbers being kept in the long term; in the author's experience, this might not always be the case, as for example, seen with the Hermann's tortoise in Spain,[16] (Albert Martinez, personal communication) with more animals in captivity than in the wild. Certainly, the reduction in exotic pets being kept will translate in a reduction of activity levels in exotic practice. Equally, if animals are kept illegally, their keepers are probably less likely to seek veterinary advice, which could negatively impact the welfare of those animals. Traditionally, the approach in the European countries has been to protect native species and prohibit keeping them as pets, contrary to other countries such as Australia, which do the opposite; the rationale behind the first approach focuses in stopping poaching, while the second one aims to avoid the introduction of invasive species. Both can cause a significant damage on the local biodiversity, and the direction taken is likely mostly influenced by previous experiences.

Positive List Approach: The legislation following this model provides a list of the animals that are allowed to be kept as pets; only the animals on the list can be kept, excluding everything else. Countries such as Germany and the Netherlands embrace the positive list approach in regulating exotic pets, which extends beyond the welfare of individual animals to encompass environmental concerns. The positive list model involves a comprehensive evaluation of species, considering not only their suitability as pets but also their potential impact on ecosystems if released. This approach aligns with the broader goals of preventing invasive species introductions.

Negative List Approach: Countries such as Belgium and Switzerland adopt a negative list approach, explicitly stating which species are prohibited as pets. This regulatory model not only addresses the potential dangers associated with certain exotic animals but also contributes to preventing the unintentional release of invasive species into the wild. By restricting ownership to approved species, these countries mitigate the risk of pets becoming invasive and causing ecological harm. The European Union, and the UK after Brexit, recognizing the ecological risks posed by invasive species, have implemented legislation specifically targeting the introduction and spread of these species. The European Union (EU) has a comprehensive framework, the Regulation (EU) No 1143/2014, which aims to prevent, minimize, and mitigate the adverse impacts of invasive alien species on biodiversity and ecosystems. Member states are required to take measures to manage and control invasive species listed in the regulation.

There are multiple factors contributing to the legal changes, reflecting the cultural changes the different European societies are experiencing, and their values regarding animals. Unfortunately, as in many other aspects, society seems to be extremely polarized in the topic, making it difficult to find middle grounds for the professionals influenced from the different involved parties.

The regulation of exotic pets in European countries encompasses not only considerations for animal welfare and responsible ownership but also addresses the broader ecological implications associated with invasive species. Positive and negative list approaches, coupled with legislation targeting invasive species, should contribute to a comprehensive framework aimed at safeguarding biodiversity and ecosystems.

Legislation and regulations about the use of medications and prescriptions, including "the cascade"

European Union legislation, applicable to all member states, establishes minimum standards. While individual member states may enact more stringent national legislation, they are prohibited from diminishing these established standards.

Generally speaking, the vast majority of medication used in exotic practice is used "off license," as only a handful of medications are licensed for exotic pets; a few medications are commercially available for commonly kept exotic pets, but the majority of medications are targeted for small companion animals or farm animals. Exotic formularies[18],[19] facilities adequate and safe use of medications in the wide range of species seen.

The European Union (EU) also plays a role in harmonizing veterinary medicine regulations across its member states, through the European Medicines Agency (EMA), a key regulatory body at the EU level that evaluates and authorizes veterinary medicines. However, each country in Europe can have its own regulations and authorities overseeing veterinary medicines.

In recent years, a few countries have explored and/or considered further changes to their legislation to regulate veterinary medications; for example, France explored the possibility of stopping veterinary practices from directly supplying medications, which was finally not approved.

The Regulation (EU) 2019/6 is a legislative framework established by the European Union (EU) concerning veterinary medicinal products. Enforced since January 28, 2022, the regulation aims to enhance the functioning of the internal market for veterinary medicines, ensuring the availability of safe and effective veterinary drugs while promoting innovation. Key elements include the centralization of marketing authorization procedures, fostering competition, addressing antimicrobial resistance, and emphasizing pharmacovigilance to monitor the safety of veterinary medicinal products throughout their lifecycle. The regulation contributes to harmonizing veterinary medicine regulations across EU member states for better animal health and welfare.

In the UK, there is special regulations about the prescription of medication, known as the "Cascade" particularly relevant for exotic practice, given the extremely limited number of licensed products available. The Cascade is a risk-based decision-tree to help veterinary surgeons decide which product to use when there is no authorized veterinary medicine available.[17] The Cascade facilitates and guides the used of nonlicensed products, with a 5 steps Table (**Table 1**).

It is also required that the client must be informed about the off licences used, and a signed consent obtained, prior to the prescription of off licence medications. Equally important is to keep records of it; The RCVS could seek clarification and why and how the medications are prescribed off license. The clinician could also be asked and is expected to be doing an evidence based, choice, balancing the risks and benefits of using an off license medication, including in the decision making process the animal, the owner, the person administering the medicine, consumers of produce from treated animals which may contain residues of the veterinary medicine, the environment and the wider public health (ie antibiotic resistance).

The COVID-19 pandemic

The COVID-19 pandemic has had a significant impact on the pet industry, influencing various aspects from pet ownership trends to supply chain dynamics. With lockdowns

Table 1	
The 5 steps to follow when prescribing medications by veerinary surgeons practicing in Great Britain	
Step	**Permitted Source**
Step 1[a]	Veterinary medicine with a Marketing Authorization valid in GB or UK wide for indicated species and condition
Step 2	Veterinary medicine with a Marketing Authorization valid in NI for indicated species and condition, in accordance with a Special Import Certificate from the VMD is required
Step 3	Veterinary medicine with a Marketing Authorization valid in GB, NI or UK wide for a different species or condition. For products not authorized in GB or UK wide a Special Import Certificate from the VMD is required
Step 4	Human medicine with a Marketing Authorization valid in GB, NI or UK wide OR an authorized veterinary medicine from outside of the UK. For products not authorized in GB or UK wide a Special Import Certificate from the VMD is required; in the case of a food-producing animal the medicine must be authorised in a food-producing species
Step 5	Extemporaneous preparation prepared by a vet, pharmacist or person holding an appropriate Manufacturer's Authorization, located in the UK
Exception	In exceptional circumstances, a human medicine may be imported from outside of the UK. For products not authorized in GB or UK wide a Special Import Certificate from the VMD is required

[a] Please note this differs slightly in Northern Ireland.

and social distancing measures in place, some services were temporarily halted or adjusted to adhere to safety protocols. One of the most notorious effects that the pandemic and the lockdowns experienced in different countries was initially on the workforce. In many countries, veterinarians were considered essential workers, and could continue to provide at least emergency care. The approached taken differed across countries, companies, and veterinary practices, but overall, most "routine" consults were put on whole, at least initially. However, most of the consultations within exotic pet medicine are not considered routine, compared with small animal practice. The reduction of colleagues working, with a similar amount of work, caused an impact on the exotic veterinary practices, many of whom took months, of not years, to recover.

The companionship offered by pets became particularly appealing during times of uncertainty, leading to increased adoption rates across various regions. With more people working from home, there was an increased interest in having pets as companions. Many people turned to pet acquisition,[7] either by adoption or buying, during lockdowns and periods of social isolation, further contributing to the mentioned problematic by increasing the demand for veterinary care.

The heightened awareness of health and well-being during the pandemic extended to pets. This led to increased interest in high-quality pet food, supplements, and veterinary care, with owners placing a greater emphasis on the overall health of their animals. The pandemic accelerated the shift toward online shopping, including the pet industry. Online pet retail and e-commerce platforms experienced increased demand for pet supplies, food, and accessories as people sought convenient ways to care for their pets without visiting physical stores.

Cost of living crisis and Ukraine war

Following the previously mentioned situation, with an increased demand of veterinary services and over-stretched workforce in the veterinary industry as a whole (including the exotic pet practice), the different European countries have experienced, to different degrees, the so called "cost of living crisis." The cost-of-living crisis is a complex issue influenced by a combination of economic, social, and geopolitical factors, including the inflation, the supply chain disruptions, the rising energy prices, wage stagnations, housing costs, global economic condition, recent geopolitical events, and natural disasters, which ultimately has caused an generalized increase in prices of goods and services, but might not have equality manifested in the average income of European salaries.

THE COST-OF-LIVING CRISIS HAS HAD BOTH DIRECT AND INDIRECT EFFECTS ON EXOTIC PET KEEPING

Direct Cost Impact: Exotic pets often require specialized care, including specific diets, enclosures, and veterinary care. The cost of maintaining these requirements can be relatively high. In times of economic hardship, individuals and families may reconsider or reduce discretionary spending, including expenses related to exotic pets. This could lead to challenges in providing the necessary care for these animals, and has ultimately cause a significant increase on abandonment and request for the rehoming of pets, exacerbated in exotic pets, as often the prevision of adequate husbandry requires the use of energy, unlike traditional pets.

Indirect Impact: Economic difficulties may also affect the pet trade and breeding industries. Breeding and supplying exotic pets involve costs, and if the demand for these pets decreases due to economic constraints, it may impact those involved in breeding and selling exotic animals.

Legal and Regulatory Changes: Economic challenges might also prompt governments to reassess and potentially change regulations related to exotic pet keeping. Stricter regulations could be introduced to ensure the welfare of exotic animals, or there may be changes to licensing and permitting processes.

CLIENT EXPECTATIONS/ACCESS TO INTERNET

The widespread availability and access to the internet have significantly transformed various aspects of society, including the field of veterinary services. The ability of pet owners to access information at their fingertips has led to both positive and challenging consequences for client education and expectations within the veterinary industry.

With the advent of the internet, pet owners now have unparalleled access to a vast array of information related to animal health, care, and veterinary practices. Websites, forums, and social media platforms provide a platform for individuals to share experiences, seek advice, and gather information on pet-related topics. This democratization of information can empower pet owners, allowing them to be more informed about their pets' health and well-being; moreover, the internet has enhanced communication between veterinarians and clients. Online platforms serve as channels for clients to engage with veterinary professionals, seek clarification, and receive guidance. This improved communication fosters a collaborative relationship, whereby clients and veterinarians can work together to ensure the best possible care for the animals.

However, while access to information is no longer limited, the current challenge nowadays is filtering and selecting the correct information, and in the recent years, the ability of differentiating between objective, unbiased information and biased (or simply incorrect) sources. The abundance of online information also presents challenges in managing client expectations. Some pet owners may attempt self-diagnosis based on information found online, leading to potential misinformation and misunderstandings. Additionally, exposure to success stories or miraculous cures on the internet may contribute to unrealistic expectations regarding treatment effectiveness and outcomes. There is a risk of clients overrelying on online advice, potentially bypassing professional veterinary guidance and delaying necessary care. Striking a balance between the valuable information available online and the expertise of veterinary professionals becomes essential to ensure the well-being of animals.

CORPORATES IN THE VET INDUSTRY

The veterinary industry has undergone a significant transformation in recent years, marked by the increasing presence of corporate entities. The veterinary industry in Europe has traditionally been dominated by independent practices, but the influx of corporate players has brought about both opportunities and challenges, particularly affecting exotic pet veterinary care.

Corporate entry into the veterinary sector has been driven by various factors, including economies of scale, enhanced resources, and standardized practices. Large corporate entities can leverage their size to negotiate better deals on supplies, invest in advanced technology, and establish standardized procedures across multiple locations. This shift has the potential to improve overall efficiency and standardization in veterinary care.

However, the impact of corporate involvement is nuanced, with implications for exotic pet practice. Exotic pet care often requires specialized knowledge and equipment, and independent practices have historically been at the forefront of providing such expertise. The corporate model, focused on streamlining operations and maximizing profit margins, may inadvertently sideline the nuanced and personalized care that exotic pets often require.

Furthermore, the corporatization of veterinary services may contribute to a more transactional approach to animal care. Exotic pet practices, which thrive on building strong relationships with clients due to the unique nature of their patients, may face challenges in maintaining the same level of personalized care under corporate structures driven by profit margins.

The corporate shift also brings changes in the employment landscape for veterinarians. While corporate entities may offer stability and benefits, they often come with productivity expectations that may affect work-life balance for veterinarians, potentially impacting their ability to provide quality care.

EDUCATION IN EXOTIC PET MEDICINE, POSTGRADUATE QUALIFICATIONS/ SPECIALIST TRAINING

In the study already mentioned, most veterinarians (54,5%) reported that exotic animal medicine had not been included at all in their veterinary studies, while the 39.5% reported they was insufficiently included in their curriculum. Barely a 6% of the participants believed that that exotic animal medicine was adequately covered in their undergraduate studies. Although these figures are a few years old, and more universities and vet schools have incorporated zoologic medicine in their courses, it remains an area for significant improvement in European teaching institutions.

Different levels of postgraduate training, as well as qualifications, exist. Not all European countries currently recognizes in their laws and regulations the figure of the veterinary specialists, widely understood in the profession as those who have obtained a diploma and are board certified. In Europe, the European Board of Veterinary Specialization (EBVS) includes under its umbrella the European College of Zoologic Medicine (ECZM) as the college focused in zoologic medicine, including exotic pet medicine. The college has currently 5 different specialities, some taxa-based, while two are based on the area of work. The number of recognised specialists are relatively small, representing less than 6% of the total of recognized specialist (228/4000). Some European countries already had their own system prior to the appearance of the ECZM, but the numbers of specialists within the field might not necessarily be proportionally higher; for example, in France, within the recognized specialist, only 0.4% are specialists in Zoo and NAC.[20]

Other postgraduate qualifications, which sit in between the general practitioner and the specialists, include the certificates provided by different organizations, institutions, or companies.[21]

DISCLOSURE

No conflict of interest.

REFERENCES

1. EU Positive List, Eurogroup for Animals, Available at: https://www.eurogroupfor animals.org/files/eurogroupforanimals/2023-03/2023_03_efa_EU%20Positive% 20List_White%20Paper.pdf. [Accessed December 20, 2023].

2. Irving-Pease EK, Frantz LAF, Sykes N, et al. Rabbits and the specious origins of domestication. Trends Ecol Evol 2018. https://doi.org/10.1016/j.tree.2017.12.009. Available at: https://qmro.qmul.ac.uk/xmlui/handle/123456789/34474.

3. Available at: https://www.google.com/search?q=Nouveaux+Animaux+de+Compagnie&rlz=1C5CHFA_enGB958GB959&oq=Nouveaux+Animaux+de+Compagnie&gs_lcrp=EgZjaHJvbWUyBggAEEUYOdIBBzI3N2owajeoAgCwAgA&sourceid=chrome&ie=UTF-8#:~:text=Le%20bien%2D%C3%AAtre,et%2Dla%2Dprotection%2D. [Accessed December 20, 2023].

4. Order of August 11, 2006 establishing the list of species, breeds or varieties of domestic animals, LegiFrance, Available at: https://www.legifrance.gouv.fr/jorf/id/JORFTEXT000000789087. [Accessed December 20, 2023].

5. What are new companion animals or NAC? EOC, Available at: https://eoc.cat/nuevos-animales-de-compania-nac/. [Accessed December 20, 2023].

6. PDSA Animal Wellbeing Paw Report 2023: Available at: https://www.pdsa.org.uk/what-we-do/pdsa-animal-wellbeing-report/paw-report-2023/pet-populations#:~:text=In%202023%2C%2053%25%20of%20UK,UK%20adults%20owned%20a%20dog.

7. UK Pet Population, UK Pet food, Available at: https://www.ukpetfood.org/information-centre/statistics/uk-pet-population.html. [Accessed December 20, 2023].

8. De Briyne N., Challenges seen with treatment of exotic pets in veterinary practice exotic pets in veterinary practice, Available at: https://www.researchgate.net/publication/333002661_Challenges_Seen_with_Treatment_of_Exotic_Pets_in_Veterinary_Practice_Exotic_Pets_in_Veterinary_Practice. [Accessed December 20, 2023].

9. The Long Eurasian Journey of Ancient and Medieval Veterinary Medicine, CGCPVE, Available at: https://www.colvet.es/es/24-Publicaciones/51-Historia/22-El-Largo-viaje-euroasiatico-de-la-veterinaria-antigua-y-medieval.htm. [Accessed December 20, 2023].

10. Elizabeth Street Veterinary Clinic, Available at: https://www.esvc.co.uk/index.php/history-blog/65-is-the-esvc-the-oldest-veterinary-facility-in-the-uk-2. [Accessed December 20, 2023].

11. Veterinary Medicine, Available at: https://en.wikipedia.org/wiki/Veterinary_medicine#cite_note-8. [Accessed December 20, 2023].

12. Find a Vet Practice, Available at: https://findavet.rcvs.org.uk/find-a-vet-practice/?filter-keyword=&filter-searchtype=practice&treated9=true. [Accessed December 20, 2023].

13. Association of Exotic Mammal Veterinarians, Available at: https://aemv.site-ym.com/search/custom.asp?id=6650. [Accessed December 20, 2023].

14. Association of Avian Veterinarians, Available at: https://www.aav.org/search/newsearch.asp. [Accessed December 20, 2023].

15. Halbwax M., Addressing the illegal wildlife trade in the European Union as a public health issue to draw decision makers attention, Available at: https://www.ncbi.nlm.nih.gov/pmc/articles/PMC7550130/. [Accessed December 20, 2023].

16. Mediterranean turtle, Gencat, Available at: https://mediambient.gencat.cat/es/05_ambits_dactuacio/patrimoni_natural/fauna-autoctona-protegida/gestio-especies-protegides-amenacades/reptils/tortuga_mediterrania/. [Accessed December 20, 2023].

17. Veterinary medicine Guidance Note, Veterinary medicines Doctorate, Available at: https://assets.publishing.service.gov.uk/media/5a817bfeed915d74e623283f/VMGNote13.PDF. [Accessed December 20, 2023].

18. Hedley J. BSAVA Small Animal Formulary 11th Edition, Part B: Exotic Pets. British Small Animal Veterinary Association; 2023.
19. Beaufrére H, Welle KR, et al. Birds. In: Carpenter JW, Harms CA, editors. Carpenter's exotic animal formulary. Sixth edition. Elsevier; 2022. p. 223–44.
20. Atlas démographique de la profession vétérinaire 2021. Available at: https://www.veterinaire.fr/system/files/files/2021-11/ODV-ATLAS-NATIONAL-2021.pdf. [Accessed December 20, 2023]
21. https://www.esavs.eu/; https://improveinternational.com/

Exotic Animal Practice in Mexico, Central, and South America

Enrique Yarto-Jaramillo, DVM[a], Jorge Rivero, MVZ[b],
Irindi Çitaku, LMV[c],*

KEYWORDS

- Latin America • Exotic pet practice • Development of exotic pet medicine
- History of exotic pets in Latin America

KEY POINTS

- Exotic animal medicine in Latin America (LATAM) has seen significant development with Mexico, Brazil, and Argentina leading the way in offering resources, training programs, and a large number of specialists in various areas of veterinary medicine, including exotic animals.
- The survey conducted in LATAM revealed that 43.5% of practitioners work or own exotic-pet only practices, while 56.5% practice at mixed-species clinics or hospitals, with 52% of clinics having 2 or more exotic veterinaries.
- Access to medication for exotic animals is a challenge in many LATAM countries with limited resources for public institutions compared to private practices, which can set up technology at their will and possibilities.
- The future of exotic clinics in LATAM requires more educational opportunities, practical courses, and the implementation of conferences, virtual and in-person courses, certifications, and externships endorsed by accredited organizations/institutions and universities.

INTRODUCTION

Latin America (LATAM) comprises from Mexico to Argentina, whereas Mexico is geographically part of North America. Central America includes 7 countries from north at the border with Mexico to south at the border with South America: Guatemala, Belize, El Salvador, Honduras, Nicaragua, Costa Rica, and Panama. Additionally, the subcontinent South America encompasses 13 sovereign countries, which in

[a] Exotic Pets and Wildlife, Centro Veterinario México, Augusto Rodin 282, Mexico City 03730, Mexico; [b] 841 West, Camino Capria, Sahuarita, AZ 85629, USA; [c] Exotic Pets and Wildlife, Centro Veterinario México, Mexico City, Mexico
* Corresponding author. Gonzalez Calderon 18, Colonia Observatorio, 11860, Miguel Hidalgo, Mexico City, Mexico.
E-mail address: irindicitaku@yahoo.com

Vet Clin Exot Anim 27 (2024) 585–592
https://doi.org/10.1016/j.cvex.2024.03.011
1094-9194/24/© 2024 Elsevier Inc. All rights reserved.

alphabetical order are Argentina, Bolivia, Brazil, Chile, Colombia, Ecuador, Guyana, Paraguay, Peru, Suriname, the Republic of Trinidad & Tobago, Uruguay, and Venezuela. Also, 1 internal territory-the French Guiana, 2 dependent territories-South Georgia and Falkland Islands (British Overseas Territories), plus 5 dependent territories from the United States of America (USA), are considered in the south of America. However, as for this article LATAM will only include from Mexico to Argentina.[1]

Like much of the world, exotic animal medicine has had a slower start in LATAM compared to other areas or specialties of veterinary medicine. In the 1970s and 1980s, LATAM experienced a great migration of its population to larger cities.

This allowed for economic growth, which prompted many people to keep companion animals and exotic pets, plus being encompassed biogeographically within the Neotropical realm, which stands out by its flora and fauna megadiversity. Wildlife trafficking became increasingly popular and a big economic driver for many communities, besides an opportunity for many to possess wild animals as pets. This led to an increase in demand for veterinary services for exotic species.

At that time there was a very little knowledge about the care of exotic species and few scientific resources could be found. Much of the veterinary care for exotic species had to be extrapolated from human, livestock, and companion animal medicine. Unfortunately, the majority of diseases exotic animals were prone to back then and now in several places still have to do with inappropriate husbandry and lack of education regarding the basic needs of the species being kept. The 1990's saw the opening of the first exotic animal veterinary practices in some countries, or mixed practices including exotic pets as part of their services. Most countries in LATAM lacked appropriate diets, special veterinary equipment, and medications to properly care for exotic species. With the turn of the century, the advent of the internet and the ever-increasing globalization and collaboration among veterinary practitioners brought an influx of knowledge and techniques to the exotic animal practitioner of LATAM.

At the time, there is only 1 formal specialization training program in LATAM on Wildlife Medicine and Surgery, which also strongly focuses on exotic pet medicine, being offered in Mexico at the School of Veterinary Medicine of the National Autonomous University of Mexico (UNAM), the only American Veterinary Medical Association (AVMA)-accredited institution in LATAM.

This article will explore the past, present, and future of exotic animal medicine in LATAM, highlighting the fact that from the last 2 decades, there has been a very significant development of a diversity of in-person and online training programs in exotic pet medicine in LATAM lead by Mexico, Argentina, and Brazil (in Portuguese), but with an important expansion to most Spanish-speaking countries. Further, the creation and extension of massive veterinary conferences and congresses in LATAM in the last decade has also brought the diversification of scientific programs, which more often include exotic pet medicine for general practitioners and students, and more advanced programs for exotic and zoo veterinarians seeking to improve their knowledge.

CURRENT EVIDENCE

To have a broader perspective of the history, present and future of exotic pet medicine in LATAM, a list of practitioners known to offer exotic pet services either at veterinary hospitals/clinics or itinerant modality was gathered by the authors.

A survey pertaining exotic pet medicine including specific questions (**Box 1**) was sent by email allowing participants to respond at length staying away from limiting

---

Box 1
List of questions included in the survey of the history of exotic pet medicine in Latin America

1. How long ago and how was the beginning of exotic pet medicine (EPM) in your country/city?
2. Were vets working with exotics specialized in EPM or small animal, zoo animal or other species?
3. Has the above trend change or are there now specialized vets in EPM?
4. How long ago have you been working with exotics in private practice?
5. Do you practice exotic pet practice as home visits, in a private clinic or hospital, or do you refer patients if you do not have diagnostic equipment for some cases?
6. List all the exotic pet species you see in private practice (home, clinic, hospital from higher to lower incidence.
7. What type of equipment did you use at the beginning to care for exotics and which ones do you currently use in your practice? It includes microscope, X-rays, ultrasound, automated equipment for blood count and blood chemistry, inhaled anesthesia, Computed Tomography, to name a few.
8. What is your source(s) of information/updates on exotic medicine today? You can consider books, magazines (Journals), online courses, in-person courses, postgraduate studies (only Master's, Doctorate and Specialty studies are considered postgraduate).
9. Is your clinical practice exclusive to exotics or is it mixed where dogs, cats, or other species are included?
10. If yours were an exotics-only practice, how do you run your exotics clinic? Including personnel (number of people working, work shifts, 24/7 attention)?
11. Does the veterinary profession in your country have the medicines (anesthetics, analgesics, for example) for the specialized care of exotics?
12. How do you see the future of the exotic clinic in your country?
13. What technology or information is needed to advance in this field in your country?

---

or sidetracking their responses. The survey was sent to more than 50 practitioners based in LATAM, having 25e respondents from 13 countries: Argentina, Bolivia, Brazil, Chile, Colombia, Costa Rica, El Salvador, Mexico, Nicaragua, Panama, Paraguay, Peru, and Uruguay (**Fig. 1**).

Thirty to 40 years ago, veterinarians started working with basic equipment such as X-rays, microscope, and basic general surgery equipment. Some of them use to hire external services like X-rays or ultrasound if they did not own the equipment at their practice. Fifty-six percent of respondents have done or are still doing home visits due to owner request, so they refer patients as needed, mainly for diagnostics. Conversely, 40% percent of respondents work either in a clinic or hospital and rarely refer unless it is an advanced diagnostic procedure (computed tomography [CT] or MRI) or specialized surgery. Eight percent of them do have all resources including CT and MRI also available to exotic pets at their practices.

DISCUSSION
Mexico, Brazil, and Argentina

The development of exotic pet medicine in LATAM has undoubtedly been led by Argentina, Brazil, and Mexico in alphabetical order. Consequently, each one of these countries has provided different types of resources to the materialization of veterinary

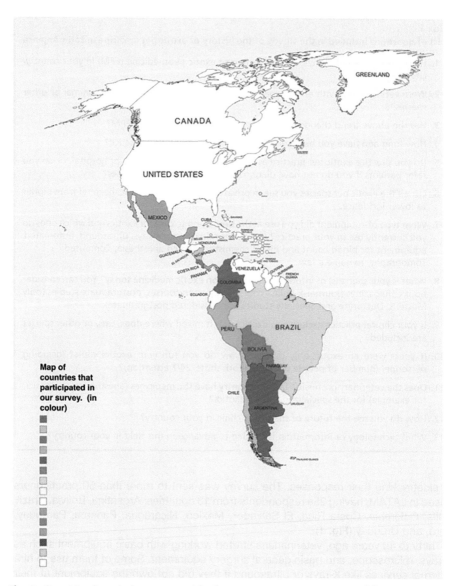

Fig. 1. Countries (in color) represented in the survey on past, present, and future of exotic pet medicine in Latin America.

medicine in LATAM including exotic pet practice starting by the fact that the 3 are the largest countries in the LATAM continent, where more schools of veterinary medicine have ever existed. Also, the economy for the last few decades, particularly in Brazil and Mexico has driven the establishment of veterinary training programs, massive scientific events, and vast number of specialists or specialized vets in diverse areas of veterinary medicine including exotic pets, becoming the target of students and practitioners from the rest of the LATAM countries seeking to be trained in nondomestic animal medicine.

In Mexico, in 1967 the first optative subject on zoo animal medicine was included in the curricula at the School of Veterinary Medicine at UNAM, Mexico, whose creator Dr Manuel Cabrera Valtierra was the first professor until 1979.

Historically, in some countries such as Mexico, Argentina, Brazil, Nicaragua and Peru zoo, circus, and wildlife veterinarians back in the 1970s and 1980s were the first practitioners consulted with exotic pets, which ranged from large cats to small birds. Other countries such as Mexico and Uruguay started offering exotic-pet only service simultaneously in 1996, either as one of its specialties at the very first 24/7 veterinary specialty hospital in LATAM, or as an exotics-only clinic, respectively.

At the time, there is only 1 program named Specialty in Wildlife Medicine and Surgery in LATAM at the School of Veterinary Medicine, at the UNAM, Mexico, currently the only AVMA accredited institution in LATAM.

Years ago, small animal, zoo, and wildlife veterinarians incorporated exotic pets in their services, but during the last 2-3 decades some respondents have gained experience from small animal/zoo animal medicine, while in some countries like Brazil and Mexico, there are specialization/postgraduate/Masters programs on wildlife and or exotic pet medicine. This has opened opportunities for betterment in exotic pet practice all over the continent.

In some countries such as Mexico, Argentina, and Brazil several training programs in nondomestic animal medicine have been offered for the last 2 decades, although post-pandemic the entire continent has experienced a tremendous rise in online courses including diplomas and short courses in exotic pet medicine and wildlife, or exotic pets only.

One veterinary hospital in Mexico City offers all the diagnostics including advanced radiology (CT, and MRI), and surgery services for exotic pets, except for radiation therapy.

Other Countries of South America

Megadiverse countries such as Colombia, Peru, Ecuador, Venezuela, and Chile have also witnessed the historical illegal possession of wildlife as pets, but which today led the legal exotic pet practice in South America after Brazil and Argentina mentioned earlier. In Colombia, domestic companion mammals, birds, reptiles, mini pigs, and other nontraditional pets are frequently seen by practitioners. Practitioners from the above-mentioned countries plus Paraguay have sought training in zoo and wildlife medicine including Conservation Medicine, being the ones treating exotic pets also, most of whom have also taken online or in-person programs locally or abroad. Some veterinaries in Colombia and elsewhere have obtained further specialization degrees in wildlife medicine including exotic pets.

Central America

Chronologically, countries in Central America have shown the overall slowest development regarding exotic pet medicine services in the continent, although most of them faced the fact of having wild animals (mostly psittacine birds, nonhuman primates, small and large exotic felids, and small native carnivores) as "exotic pets" in large numbers through the years. More recently, the trend of legal companion pets has increased in the region alike the rest of the continent, where small herbivores such as (rabbits, rodents, ferrets, and African pygmy hedgehogs), mini pigs, companion birds, and some reptile species represent the majority of veterinary patients in exotic pet services.

In most LATAM countries, back then and now, small animal (dogs and cats) clinics and hospitals have received exotic pets of all kinds during the last 30 years, but in some like Panama (2005), Nicaragua (2012), Costa Rica (2016), Bolivia (2019), and El Salvador (2021) practitioners started offering exotics-pet only service at 1 single clinic, or mixed practices.

Many practitioners from several countries in LATAM have been trained abroad through practical courses, externships, and other types of programs including clinical rotations belonging to formal university programs. Countries such as Mexico, Brazil, USA, Spain, and United Kingdom, to name a few, have been the target of Latin veterinarians to get trained in exotic pet practice.

During the last 20 years up to now, more than 40% of respondents have used X-rays, ultrasound, and inhaled anesthesia. Nowadays, up to 80% of veterinarians have their own practice offering diagnostics including automated blood machines, X-rays, ultrasound, multiparameter monitors, and inhaled anesthesia. Some 20% still rent practices to perform surgery or diagnostics, refer or call anesthetists/surgeons to perform procedures in their clinics.

Different types of information are used to update themselves by the same person, so the following are the predominant according to respondents: reference books (28%), online courses and journals (26%), post-graduate programs (Master and Doctorate) (9%), online and in-person talks and seminars (8%), and externships/internships (3%).

The overall results of our survey show 43.5% of practitioners' work or own exotic-pet only practices (**Fig. 2**), while 56.5% practice at mixed-species clinics or hospitals.

Fifty-two percent of clinics or hospitals in LATAM have 2 or more exotic veterinarians , while 48% have only 1 exotic practitioner with 1 to 4 interns in the exotic pet service.

From Mexico to Argentina, most veterinarians claim they do not have access to a good number of drugs they need on daily practice. This leads to a few options on analgesics/anesthetic drugs, plus non-existent compounding pharmacies for any other

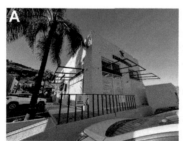
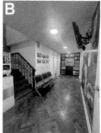
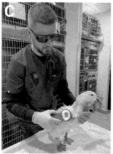
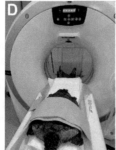
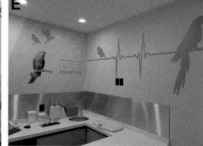

Fig. 2. Private exotic-only practices in Latin America (Queretaro, Mexico, Lima, Peru, and Mexico City). (*A*) Faunaterra, Querétaro, México; (*B*) Dr PLUMAS, Avian and Exotic Pet Clinic. Lima -Perú; (*C–E*) Centro Veterinario Mexico, Mexico City, Mexico.

therapeutic agents. In some countries opioids that are used frequently for pain management in exotic pets are unavailable and this is because veterinarians are not considered part of the health sector in LATAM. In Latin American countries, it is from hard to impossible to get the importation permits for feed stuff or drugs from abroad unless there is a formal distributor that usually is the case only for the largest veterinarymarkets based in the largest countries.

In the last few years, the exotic pet medicine practice and mostly post-coronavirus disease 2019 pandemic has gained popularity in many countries and more and more young veterinarians are focusing their profession on this area of veterinary medicine.

Nowadays, the owners are more conscious about the need of their pets and support the diagnostic route of different challenging pathologies that exotic pets present. These services are expensive most of the time in the exotic pet field and veterinarians are constantly in search of more affordable prices and easy access to diagnostic methodology for their patients.

Veterinarians in Central and most South American countries require more practical courses (**Fig. 3**) in their countries as source of updating and hands-on practice, although at least a number of online and in-person courses are available in the area.

FUTURE CONSIDERATIONS

In the author's opinion, the following steps are necessary to improve exotic practice in LATAM. Veterinarians in LATAM need more educational opportunities to further their knowledge. First off, this should start by changing/complementing the curricula of the majority of schools of veterinary medicine, which in terms of exotic pet medicine is from non-existent to really scarce in most countries and universities. Furthermore,

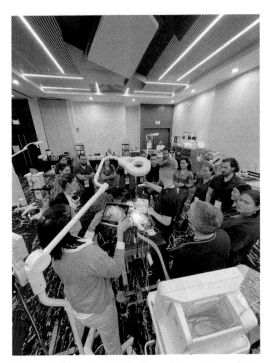

Fig. 3. In-person training program in exotic pet medicine, Costa Rica.

this can be achieved through the implementation of conferences, virtual and in-person courses, certifications, and externships endorsed by accredited organizations/institutions and universities in most countries.

Exotic pet veterinarians should have high-level educational opportunities in their native language, Spanish. Further, to be classified as a legitimate specialist in exotic animal practice the formation of a Diplomate program with appropriate testing should be considered. To assist veterinarians in supporting the health care of exotic animals, most LATAM countries need access to appropriate products and high-quality commercial diets. Large companies should expand business to LATAM countries, although bureaucracy and heterogeneity of laws and policies in each country have delayed this fact. Without access to proper nutrition and husbandry, the practice of exotic animal medicine has too many challenges.

In some countries, it is difficult to find necessary medications. The exotic practitioner community needs to come together to lobby regulatory boards to allow easier access to medication in exotic animals.

As new technology and techniques become available, veterinary practices in LATAM should have the opportunity and equal access for acquiring them. However, this is not always feasible since resources for public institutions do not equal private practices, which set up technology at their will and possibilities.

Finally, we believe all veterinarians who share an interest in exotic animal practice would benefit from having easier access to membership in critical exotic practice organizations such as the Association of Avian Veterianrians, Association of Exotic Mammal Veterinarians, Associaton of Reptiles and Amphibian Veterianrians and American Association of Fish Veterinarians, albeit some of them do offer special rates to practitioners from developing nations. Veterinarians also need to become an active part of their own local exotic/wildlife practice associations to be an active part of professional groups of like-minded people. As the world becomes increasingly connected, it is important for exotic animal peers to network and share information to better support the health and conservation of the exotic species we all take care of.[2,3]

ACKNOWLEDGMENTS

We deeply thank our peers all along Latin America for participating in our survey: Argentina: Pedrosa F., Settembrini J., Sciabarrasi A., Di Nucci D.; Chile: Crisosto S., Dunner C.; Bolivia: Mendez S.; Peru: Canales S., Coronado J.; Mexico: Lewy C., Alonso M., Martinez A., Arce I., Fuantos A.; Panama: Reyes J.; Costa Rica: Rusz L.; Paraguay: Vetter R., Pesole D.; Brazil: Couto E., Fonseca C.; Uruguay: Infante P.; Colombia: Ariza A., Jaramillo N.; Nicaragua: Molina C.; El Salvador: Soriano K.

DISCLOSURE

Nothing to disclose.

REFERENCES

1. Countries in Latin America & the Caribbean. Available at: http://lanic.utexas.edu/subject/countries/.
2. Yarto-Jaramillo E, Soares-Neto LL. Latin American zoo veterinarian associations. Elsevier; 2023. p. 25–8.
3. Speer BL, Olsen GP, Doneley B, et al. Common conditions of commonly held companion birds in multiple parts of the world. Elsevier; 2016. p. 777–94.

Dungeons and Dragons
Culture Differences in Attitudes Toward Exotic Animals

Shangzhe Xie, BSc/BVMS, MVS, PhD, DABVP (Avian Practice), DACCM[a],*,
Ji Zhen Low, BSc/BVMS, PGCert VetEd, FHEA[b]

KEYWORDS

• Culture • Exotic animal practice • Veterinary medicine

KEY POINTS

• The views and attitudes toward exotic animal species are constantly evolving and may eventually converge in the way that cats and dogs are now widely accepted as part of most societies around the world.
• The choice and popularity of exotic animal species as pets is a complex interaction of many different factors, including legislation and availability.
• Despite the consistent portrayal of rabbits serving multiple roles across different cultures, they appear to have established themselves as predominantly a pet species, to the point that they form the majority of the caseload in many exotic animal practices around the world.
• If cultural depictions were to be the main driving factor behind people's choices of exotic pets, then exotic animal species representing the dragon should be more popular in Chinese/eastern cultures that revere the dragon, but it seems likely that people's choices of exotic pet species are driven more by practicality and ease of obtaining and caring for the animal.
• Media, as the representation of modern popular culture, is often thought to be a factor too, but there has been very little evidence to demonstrate this.

EXOTIC ANIMAL PRACTICE AROUND THE WORLD

As demonstrated in the rest of this issue, the way exotic animals are viewed around the world differ. These views and attitudes are constantly evolving and may eventually converge in the way that cats and dogs are now widely accepted as part of most societies around the world. However, this speed of evolution may depend on how entrenched some of these attitudes are, and this is in turn potentially dependent on

[a] Veterinary Health, Mandai Wildlife Group, 80 Mandai Lake Road, Singapore; [b] School of Applied Science, Temasek Polytechnic, 21 Tampines Avenue 1, Singapore
* Corresponding author.
E-mail address: shangzhe.xie@mandai.com

Vet Clin Exot Anim 27 (2024) 593–600
https://doi.org/10.1016/j.cvex.2024.03.002

the origins of these attitudes. While recognizing the importance of not over-generalizing cultural practices within or between cultural and racial groups, the authors have utilized their cultural experiences as ethnic Chinese growing up in cosmopolitan Singapore and life experiences studying and working in Australia, New Zealand, and United States to explore the effect of culture on exotic animal practice using 3 groups of animals as examples. These species were chosen based on the Chinese zodiac, with it being the year of the Dragon at the point of writing and publication, the year of the Rabbit prior, and the year of the Snake following.

DOES CULTURE SHAPE ATTITUDES IN EXOTIC ANIMAL PRACTICE?

The importance of cultural competence of veterinarians is an area of growing traction and consequently, there is increasing awareness of the importance of including this within veterinary curricula.[1] There is general consensus that cultural influence can have far-reaching effects as cultural beliefs and norms can impact what is considered acceptable practice and effective communication.[2]

Even with this recognition, there are very few studies specific to veterinarians. A recent study from Hong Kong indicating that shared decision making was valued by clients and could minimize client conflict only sampled western-trained vets.[3] The vets' amount of working experience in Hong Kong was not specified, and it is possible that a biased population was sampled.

Human medicine literature covers this topic better. There is a published Southeast Asian communication guideline for doctors,[4] and even though it is nuanced for the local Indonesian culture, it adopted a similar framework as the patient consultation process in the Calgary-Cambridge model from which the veterinary guideline was derived.[5] The Southeast Asian communication guideline concurs with studies from human health care and veterinary literature of Western and Asian origin[6] that core communication skills such as empathy,[7] trust, and rapport,[8] and appropriate non-verbal cues[9] are key.

Anecdotally, from a recent class in Singapore discussing client conflict manage-ment that required veterinary technician students to use ChatGPT for generating and analyzing phrases for suitability for diffusing difficult situations, students identi-fied core skills such as empathy, active listening, and tone of voice important aspects of communication. While this experience indicated that the western approach to communication training seemed to yield the same results even for students in an Asian culture, thereby transcending culture, it does not support the assumption that communication in Asia is different from western culture.[10] The only point of dif-ference that students pointed out was that the use of the Singlish (slang for Singapor-ean English) vernacular was something they had observed to be prevalent and therefore something that they would include in their client interactions. Students explained that Singlish made the conversation feel natural and familiar, conveying a common language that fostered the development of rapport with clients. Singapore is a multiracial nation with 4 main races, each with their own languages and dialects. Although English remains the first language of Singapore, many people, particularly the older generations, may converse in their ethnic language or dialect more fluently. Of course, becoming multilingual is not feasible for most, and this has surfaced an interesting challenge of the language barrier which is recognized in Singapore nurse–patient communication,[6] a recurring theme in Asian veterinary literature too.[3] In the cultural context of Singapore, therefore, the common Singlish vernacular could potentially be a unifying factor that could transcend race, alleviating a potentially major barrier to client communication.

In many cultures, doctors are often considered to be at the top of the medical hierarchy and highly respected by patients.[4] Based upon some of the available literature from Asian nations such as Indonesia, Pakistan,[11] and Malaysia,[12] this is said to be contributed by patients who may be less educated in the countries studied, further widening the disparity in hierarchy. This phenomenon is possibly more ubiquitous than these authors have alluded to. In a developed nation like Singapore where the vast majority of the population are well-educated, studies of human nurses still echo the sentiments of a hierarchical structure.[13] From the authors' experiences in clinical practice, it was clear that there is a perceived disparity in the way clients regard veterinarians and veterinary technicians. Phrases such as "can you double check with the vet?" and "I think I'll just wait for the vet" were commonplace in Australia, United States, and Singapore.

Other than the effects of cultural differences in the way veterinary medicine is practiced in general, the way the animal being presented by the client at a veterinary practice is perceived may also differ among cultures. One study suggests that the affordability may be an important factor that influences the level of veterinary care provided for dogs and cats and this is despite the fact that owners considered their pets as family.[14] Species that are traditionally considered domestic animals, for example, dogs, cats, cattle, horses, have evolved culturally at different paces in different parts of the world. The concept of a dog being "part of the family" is more established in some cultures than others. Given the wide range of exotic animal species that are kept as pets, this difference in pace of evolution is even more pronounced, and the following examples will demonstrate this phenomenon.

THE RABBIT

Depending on the culture, rabbits can be viewed as pets, pests, or food animals. One particular encounter in exotic animal practice in Australia demonstrated the importance in establishing this upfront during client interactions. A client with a European accent had requested a phone consult as he noticed one of his rabbits had developed swollen eyelids, and the veterinarian (one of the authors) proceeded to explain that this was likely a clinical sign of myxomatosis. The consult went into a detailed explanation of etiology, lack of specific treatment options, and poor prognosis for the patient. There was a brief moment of silence after the long explanation, and the client responded with: "All I wanted to know was whether it is safe to eat this rabbit".

Even when viewed as a food animal, the way rabbits are perceived differ within South Africa, where ethnicity affects whether people believe that rabbits were unclean, for the poor, and/or unhealthy.[15] Similar differences also exist in Italy, where rabbits have multiple roles of equal significance.[16] Rabbits are also popular characters in folklores and children's stories, which may affect the way they are viewed by people growing up with those stories. In the story associated with the Mid-Autumn Festival in Chinese culture, the main protagonist Chang Er ascended to the moon with the rabbit as her companion. While this may inspire some to desire a rabbit as a pet, confectionary made in the shape of rabbits are also commercially sold during the festival to be consumed. Similarly, many children in western culture grow up with the stories of Peter Rabbit and his friends. It is very common for pet rabbits in these cultures to be named after characters of this series. While this serves as a motivation for children in these cultures to ask for a rabbit as their first pet, many stories also revolve around rabbits wreaking havoc on the farmer's vegetable patch or escaping from predators. However, these other roles of the rabbits in these stories do not seem to contribute to them being viewed in a negative light as pests or food animals.

Despite the consistent portrayal of rabbits serving multiple roles across different cultures, they appear to have established themselves as predominantly a pet species, to the point that they form the majority of the caseload in many exotic animal practices around the world.

THE DRAGON

The dragon is viewed in stark contrast between Chinese/eastern and western cultures.[17–19] The Chinese dragon is viewed overwhelmingly in the positive light, with ancient Chinese emperors, idioms and stories painting them as symbols of auspicious and good luck. Although they are sometimes the villain in stories for the hero to defeat, they are more often a source of strength and help in times of need, for example, in Mulan. The form usually depicted is one with a long, slender body covered with elaborate scales and a head with intricate features. Their limbs are usually short, and lack any true functional value, given that they can usually fly in the absence of wings. This is very similar in other eastern cultures, for example, Vietnamese and Japanese.[20]

On the other hand, the western dragon is more commonly the villain, and associated with death and destruction,[17–19] for example, smaug in Lord of the Rings and other dragons that are used to guard castles. The friendly dragon in Shrek was one of the few positively viewed characters, and even she was initially thought to be the guardian of the castle that needed to be slain. The western dragon usually has a larger, dinosaur-like body, with longer and more functional limbs. They are also usually depicted with wings, even though the size of these wings is disproportionately small compared to the body, and if real-world biomechanics were to apply, should not be able to propel their large bodies in flight. Most western dragons can also breathe fire, which allows them to rain destruction on a large scale.

Of course, the dragon is a mythical creature, and therefore impossible to be kept as an exotic pet. However, many reptilian species have "dragon" in their common name, for example, bearded dragon, Chinese water dragon, while others bear a resemblance in form, for example, axolotl. However, these exotic animals seem to be more popular in western countries, despite the negative connotations associated with dragons in these cultures. If cultural depictions were to be the main driving factor behind people's choices of exotic pets, then these species should be more popular in Chinese/eastern cultures that revere the dragon. Therefore, it seems likely that people's choices of exotic pet species are driven more by practicality and ease of obtaining and caring for the animal.

THE SNAKE

Compared to the dragon, the snake is more unequivocal among different cultures in its perception. Even in religious texts, the snake embodies the ultimate form of evil. Interestingly, it is possible that these texts could be referring to the "dragon" in some of these references to the "snake," as the lack of a word for "dragon" in ancient Hebrew makes it confusing to interpret texts in its original language.[17] However, as most of the translations seem able to distinguish the "snake" from the "dragon" within the same text, the snake has taken on a more distinct role in most modern cultures.

Despite these negative connotations, snakes are still relatively popular as exotic pets. They are arguably easier to care for than many mammalian or avian exotic pet species, with most of the work going into the initial set-up to ensure appropriate husbandry. Subsequent day-to-day care is then a simpler matter of ensuring appropriate husbandry including hygiene and nutrition at the right frequency. However, the ease of obtaining snakes for keeping as pets differ based on the legislation.

Venomous snakes are usually very difficult to obtain for such purposes, while even non-venomous snakes may not be allowed as pets in many jurisdictions. Given the dynamics between demand and supply in driving the speed of change of legislations, the speed of evolution of these legislations and the popularity of snakes as pets take on a "chicken and egg" relationship, that is, if snakes were legally allowed as pets, then their popularity will increase, but if there is a demand for more snakes to be kept as pets, then there will be pressure for the legislation to be changed to allow for that.

Converse to the ubiquitous negative views of the snake across cultures, the way the beauty of snakes is viewed seems to be universal as well. In 2 similar studies performed across 7 continents, there were strong cross-cultural similarities among different cultures when assessing the esthetics of snakes.[21,22] There is suggestion from these studies that Europeans (as represented by participants from Czech Republic in the study) may differ in their opinion of snakes compared to other cultures due to the lack of direct encounters with snakes and a reliance on media depiction of snakes to shape their opinions.[21,22] Compared to the dragon, which is a mythical animal that can be depicted in any way possible based on infinite artistic freedom, snakes can be portrayed in both fictional and non-fictional media. While there is possibly a shift in fictional media in featuring snakes in a more positive light, for example, focusing on the desirable characteristics of the Slytherin house in the Harry Potter series, albeit only coming across more strongly toward the end of the series, non-fictional media can also contribute in shifting the public perception of the snake. For example, documentaries can focus on the ecological contributions of snakes and the effects of climate change on snake populations. Similarly, news stories of human–snake interactions can also focus on the plight of the snakes resulting from human encroachment into their habitats, rather than sensationalizing the human deaths and injuries that sometimes arise from these interactions.

THE FUTURE

As demonstrated by the examples mentioned earlier and other studies in this issue, the choice and popularity of exotic animal species as pets is a complex interaction of many different factors. Legislation may be a strong factor, as most pet owners will not be willing to break the law in order to own an exotic pet. Availability of exotic animal species as pets are also strongly driven by legislation, either directly by law-abiding pet shops and breeders, or indirectly by the increased cost of bypassing legal channels to breed and obtain these species.

Media, as the representation of modern popular culture, is often thought to be a factor too, but there has been very little evidence to demonstrate this. There has been minimal quantitative evidence to show that there were increases in import and export of wild-caught fish in the 18 months after release of "Finding Nemo," suggesting a lack of "Nemo effect" in making aquarium fish more popular pets after watching the movie.[23] This is in contrast to the potential positive impacts movies may have on attitudes toward biodiversity conservation,[24] possibly indicating that opposition to the use of exotic animal species in popular media for fear of encouraging their popularity as pets and thereby affecting their conservation in the wild may be unfounded.

Therefore, if culture were to be considered, the cumulation of decades and centuries of public opinion as shaped by media through those times, then it should not be surprising that culture ultimately has very little influence on people's choices of exotic animal species as pets. The availability of veterinarians who can advise and treat these species may be a stronger factor in the decision-making process of pet owners deciding to obtain an exotic pet. The lack of exotic pet veterinarians in many parts of the world is a recurring theme through the other studies in this issue and may be a limiting factor in the growth of the exotic pet industry, whether in the maintenance of sustainable breeding of these species, or the willingness of legislators to allow the keeping of these pets without assurance that there was sufficient veterinary support.

The lack of exotic pet veterinarians ultimately originates from the lack of emphasis on veterinary education in this field at all levels of the industry, starting from universities. This is unlikely to change until the accreditation bodies increase the weightage of exotic animal practice in the curriculum requirements of veterinary degrees, which is unlikely to change until exotic animal species match the popularity of dogs and cats as pets. Some cultures may get to this state in the near future, while others appear to be further behind in the process. Regardless of the geographic location and cultural context of the region, exotic animal practice appears to be an area of veterinary practice that is on the rise, so stay tuned for the exciting developments of exotic animal practice around the world.

CLINICS CARE POINTS

- The views and attitudes toward exotic animal species are constantly evolving and may eventually converge in the way that cats and dogs are now widely accepted as part of most societies around the world.
- The choice and popularity of exotic animal species as pets is a complex interaction of many different factors, including legislation and availability.
- Despite the consistent portrayal of rabbits serving multiple roles across different cultures, they appear to have established themselves as predominantly a pet species, to the point that they form the majority of the caseload in many exotic animal practices around the world.
- If cultural depictions were to be the main driving factor behind people's choices of exotic pets, then exotic animal species representing the dragon should be more popular in Chinese/eastern cultures that revere the dragon, but it seems likely that people's choices of exotic pet species are driven more by practicality and ease of obtaining and caring for the animal.
- Media, as the representation of modern popular culture, is often thought to be a factor too, but there has been very little evidence to demonstrate this.

DISCLOSURE

The authors have nothing to disclose.

REFERENCES

1. Alvarez EE, Gilles WK, Lygo-Baker S, et al. Teaching cultural humility and implicit bias to veterinary medical students: a review and recommendation for best practices. J Vet Med Educ 2020;47(1):2–7.
2. Gongora J, van Gelderen I, Vost M, et al. Cultural competence is everyone's business: Embedding cultural competence in curriculum frameworks to advance veterinary education. J Vet Med Educ 2022;50(1):1–4.
3. Chan CK, Wong PW. Hong Kong veterinarians' encounters with client-related stress–a qualitative study. Front Vet Sci 2023;10.

4. Claramita M, Prabandari Y, Van Dalen J, et al. A guideline for doctor-patient communication more appropriate in South East Asia. Southeast Asia Medical Education Journal 2010;4(2):23–30.

5. Radford A, Stockley P, Silverman J, et al. Development, teaching, and evaluation of a consultation structure model for use in veterinary education. J Vet Med Educ 2006;33(1):38–44.

6. Tay LH, Ang E, Hegney D. Nurses' perceptions of the barriers in effective communication with inpatient cancer adults in Singapore. J Clin Nurs 2012;21(17-18): 2647–58.

7. McDermott MP, Tischler VA, Cobb MA, et al. Veterinarian–client communication skills: current state, relevance, and opportunities for improvement. J Vet Med Educ 2015;42(4):305–14.

8. Pun JKH. Comparing veterinary students' and practitioners' perceptions of communication in a bilingual context. Vet Rec 2021;189(12):e587.

9. Pun JK. An integrated review of the role of communication in veterinary clinical practice. BMC Vet Res 2020;16:1–4.

10. Pun JK, Chan EA, Wang S, et al. Health professional-patient communication practices in East Asia: An integrative review of an emerging field of research and practice in Hong Kong, South Korea, Japan, Taiwan, and Mainland China. Patient Educ Counsel 2018;101(7):1193–206.

11. Matusitz J, Spear J. Doctor-patient communication styles: A comparison between the United States and three Asian countries. J Hum Behav Soc Environ 2015; 25(8):871–84.

12. Thuraisingham C, Abd Razak SS, Nadarajah VD, et al. Communication skills in primary care settings: aligning student and patient voices. Educ Prim Care 2023;1–8.

13. Tan XW, Lopez V, Cleary M. Views of recent Singapore nursing graduates: factors influencing nurse–patient interaction in hospital settings. Contemp Nurse 2016; 52(5):602–11.

14. Kiefer V, Grogan KB, Chatfield J, et al. Cultural competence in veterinary practice. J Am Vet Med Assoc 2013;243(3):326–8.

15. Hoffman LC, Vosloo C, Nkhabutlane P, et al. Associations with rabbits and rabbit meat of three different ethnic groups in Stellenbosch, South Africa. J Consum Sci 2005;33:63–72.

16. Mazzucchelli F. The birth of a pet? The rabbit. Semiotics of Animals in Culture. Zoosemiotics 2018;2:103–18.

17. Liu Y. Cultural differences of Chinese loong and Western dragon. Stud Lit Lang 2015;10(3):40.

18. Bi W. Fear arising out of misinterpretation: cultural differences between the loong and the dragon. infacing our darkness. Manifestations of Fear, Horror and Terror 2015;163–71.

19. Meccarelli M. Discovering the Long: current theories and trends in research on the chinese dragon. Front Hist China 2021;16(1):99.

20. Nguyen NT. The symbol of the dragon and ways to shape cultural identities in Vietnam and Japan. Ho Chi Minh City, Vietnam: Harvard-Yenching Institute Working Paper Series; 2015.

21. Marešová J, Antonín K, Frynta D. We all appreciate the same animals: Cross-cultural comparison of human aesthetic preferences for snake species in Papua New Guinea and Europe. Ethology 2009;115(4):297–300.

22. Frynta D, Marešová J, Řeháková-Petrů M, et al. Cross-cultural agreement in perception of animal beauty: boid snakes viewed by people from five continents. Hum Ecol 2011;39:829–34.

23. Militz TA, Foale S. The "Nemo Effect": perception and reality of Finding Nemo's impact on marine aquarium fisheries. Fish Fish 2017;18(3):596–606.

24. Silk MJ, Crowley SL, Woodhead AJ, et al. Considering connections between Hollywood and biodiversity conservation. Conserv Biol 2018;32(3):597–606.

Moving?

Make sure your subscription moves with you!

To notify us of your new address, find your **Clinics Account Number** (located on your mailing label above your name), and contact customer service at:

Email: **journalscustomerservice-usa@elsevier.com**

800-654-2452 (subscribers in the U.S. & Canada)
314-447-8871 (subscribers outside of the U.S. & Canada)

Fax number: **314-447-8029**

Elsevier Health Sciences Division
Subscription Customer Service
3251 Riverport Lane
Maryland Heights, MO 63043

*To ensure uninterrupted delivery of your subscription, please notify us at least 4 weeks in advance of move.

ELSEVIER